*The Multiple Choice
Question in Medicine*

The Multiple Choice Question in Medicine

JOHN ANDERSON,
MB, BS, FRCP

*Academic Sub-Dean of the Medical School,
and Senior Lecturer in Medicine,
University of Newcastle upon Tyne*

*Honorary Consultant Physician,
Royal Victoria Infirmary,
Newcastle Area Health Authority (Teaching)*

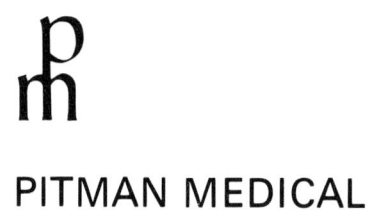

pm

PITMAN MEDICAL

First published 1976
Reprinted 1978

PITMAN MEDICAL PUBLISHING CO LTD
42 Camden Road, Tunbridge Wells,
Kent TN1 2QD

Associated Companies

UNITED KINGDOM
Pitman Publishing Ltd, London
Focal Press Ltd, London

USA
Pitman Publishing Corporation, California
Fearon Publishers Inc, California

AUSTRALIA
Pitman Publishing Pty Ltd, Melbourne

CANADA
Pitman Publishing, Toronto
Copp Clark Publishing, Toronto

EAST AFRICA
Sir Isaac Pitman and Sons Ltd, Nairobi

SOUTH AFRICA
Pitman Publishing Co SA (Pty) Ltd, Johannesburg

NEW ZEALAND
Pitman Publishing NZ Ltd, Wellington

© John Anderson, 1976

ISBN: 0 272 79376 0

Cat. No. 21 0017 81

Text set in 10/11 pt IBM Journal,
printed by photolithography, and
bound in Great Britain at The Pitman Press, Bath

Contents

Preface vi
Definition of Terms viii

1 Types of Multiple Choice Questions 1
2 Setting of Multiple Choice Questions 13
3 Candidate Responses — Lector and Opscan Sheets 23
4 Marking of Multiple Choice Questions 30
5 Evaluation of Multiple Choice Questions 40
6 Revision of Questions and Feedback 44
7 The Newcastle Computer Printout 49
8 Hints to Candidates 54

Bibliography 57

Specimen Questions 59
Breakdown of Topics 61

Indexes 148

Preface

Multiple choice questions are widely used in medical examinations but while they have now gained general acceptance as an assessment method there is still a hint of uncertainty and suspicion about the technique in some quarters. Sometimes this is because of ignorance and lack of experience, sometimes because the failings and faults of poor MCQ have been unduly emphasized, and sometimes because the examiners expect too much from them or try to use them for purposes that would be better served by some other technique. The fact remains, however, that carefully prepared MCQ are unrivalled as reliable and highly discriminatory objective tests of factual recall. At the same time higher areas of taxonomy can be assessed by means of well thought-out questions, without loss of discriminatory power.

I do not intend this to be a comprehensive theoretical review of the multiple choice question technique and its place in medical educational technology. The aim of the book is practical. The chapter headings describe the content and it is hoped that the book will be helpful to both examiners and candidates. Each group will probably concentrate on different areas although I hope that there will be something of interest for everyone in each chapter – candidates may gain reassurance as well as information from some of the more theoretical sections.

The book is very heavily biased towards the multiple true/false type of question and the Newcastle University computer program used to mark and analyse such questions. I offer no apologies for this bias – this type of question and the Newcastle program are probably used more widely in the UK than any other single format. Here it is appropriate to acknowledge the major role that Professor E. S. Page, Dr W. Anne Wood and their colleagues in the University of Newcastle Computing Laboratory have played in the evolution of MCQ techniques over the last decade or more.

There may be some repetition in the text; this is because I have attempted to make each chapter an essay complete in itself and have tried to avoid too many distracting cross-references. At the same time unnecessary repetition has been avoided by placing all the references mentioned in the text in a separate bibliography. This bibliography is not intended to be comprehensive, but refers to the more important, relevant and recent papers on the subject. The one hundred and fifty questions at the end of the book are intended as an educational as well as an assessment exercise, and comments are given on nearly all items.

If the book helps examiners to set better questions and to analyse examination results more critically, and if it assists and reassures candidates, while clarifying the technique for them, I shall be happy.

Acknowledgements

This book could not have been written without the co-operation and interest shown by Professor E. S. Page, Director of the University of Newcastle upon Tyne Computing Laboratory, and of Dr Anne Wood of the staff of the Laboratory, who has been responsible for a number of years for processing MCQ, writing appropriate programs and for seeing that the suggestions of examiners are translated from theoretical concepts into practical procedures. Miss E. D. Barraclough, Computer Manager, has also been of inestimable help over the years. I would like to acknowledge the invaluable advice and encouragement of Professor G. P. McNicol and Dr J. F. Stokes, Chairman and past Chairman respectively of the Joint Examining Board of the Royal Colleges of Physicians, and my colleagues on the Board. Over the last five years I have learnt more from them about MCQ (and about medicine) than I believed possible.

I would also like to thank Professor G. A. Smart, who introduced me to MCQ many years ago and gave me the opportunity to involve myself in a fascinating and rewarding educational experience and to Professor John N. Walton, Dean of Medicine, Mr Norman Shott, Deputy Registrar, and the Board of the Faculty of Medicine at the University of Newcastle for allowing me to refer to the Newcastle examinations and giving me permission to publish questions used in these examinations. Although I edited these questions I did not compose them all myself and I am grateful to my many colleagues who were their authors, and who continue regularly to produce questions.

Finally I would like to thank my secretary, Mrs Jacqueline Home, who typed my manuscript impeccably, my wife and family for tolerating me while the book was being prepared, and the staff of Pitman Medical for their unfailing patience and courtesy.

J. Anderson
Newcastle upon Tyne
April 1976

Definition of Terms

Confusion has arisen in the past because terms in common use in connection with MCQ mean different things to different authors. The definitions given here are those that the majority of postgraduate examining bodies, many medical schools and the University of Newcastle Computing Laboratory have found convenient.

1. A QUESTION is the basic component of a multiple choice paper. It comprises:
2. A STEM or introductory statement and a series of
3. ITEMS, identified by a letter. Items are the smallest component of the examination to which the candidate may make a response. The terms COMPLETION and ALTERNATIVE are synonymous with the term item.
4. The word STATEMENT is used at some points in this book. It really has nothing to do with MCQ and is used purely for convenience. An item may in itself be a complete statement or the stem plus an item may together make a statement. It is to this statement that the candidate responds.
5. A RESPONSE is the positive selection made by the candidate in marking the RESPONSE SHEET — whether the response be 'true', 'false' or 'do not know'. The response may be *correct* or *incorrect*, depending on whether it corresponds with the examiners' response or not. The candidate's SELECTION is in our vocabulary synonymous with his RESPONSE.
6. TRUE is *not* synonymous with CORRECT, or FALSE with INCORRECT. True and false refer to either the candidates' or the examiners' responses; by definition the examiners' responses will always be correct! The candidates' responses may be *correct* or *incorrect*.
7. The MEAN SCORE is the mean of all the candidates' scores for an individual question or for the paper as a whole.
8. 'PERCENTAGE CANDIDATES CORRECT' is exactly what it says and is given on the computer printout for each individual item.
9. An INDEX OF DISCRIMINATION may refer to a question or to an individual item and gives an indication of how well that question or item discriminates between the better and the weaker candidates. In the Newcastle Marking Program the index of discrimination is a correlation coefficient. (See Chapter 5.)

CHAPTER ONE

Types of Multiple Choice Questions

EXAMINATIONS HAVE been used since time immemorial to assess student performance, to determine whether certain standards have been achieved and to decide whether teaching objectives have been attained. One of the important functions of examinations is to rank students — the most able being graded highly and the less able being placed lower down the list. It is clearly important that such a ranked order should accurately reflect the candidates' abilities and that the grading should be as objective as possible — relying principally on performance in the examination and not depending on the foibles or idiosyncrasies of the examiners. An examination should be fair and free from examiner-bias, and the results should be influenced only by those factors that the examination is designed to test. A 'poor' examination, one that is ambiguous or one that depends more on a knowledge of the intricacies of the English language than on a knowledge of medicine, will produce results that must be interpreted with reservation.

The traditional medical examination forms include essay questions, oral confrontation and clinical and practical tests. Each form tests something different, and the subjective nature, inconsistency of marking and lack of reproducibility of these examinations (particularly essay questions) are well recognized (Smart, 1976). Nevertheless, each type still has a role to play in the assessment of undergraduates and postgraduates, always provided that the effect of examiner variability on the scores can be reduced to a minimum, and that each candidate is given a fair and equal chance of demonstrating his abilities. The objectives of any examination should be clearly defined — different forms may have different aims. It would be a sad day for medicine (and for prospective patients) if the clinical examination were to be discontinued. The oral examination, properly conducted by experienced examiners, offers a unique opportunity for the candidate to demonstrate his particular strengths, and the essay question, carefully set and assessed, allows the candidate to exhibit his ability to analyse and discuss a particular problem. The essay question that simply tests factual recall (still all too common) is as much a waste of candidate and examiner time as the oral that is used to test only factual knowledge.

During the last fifteen or more years, medical educationists have spent much time in attempting to develop methods of assessment that have been more objective, valid and fair, while indicating accurately the degree of attainment by the candidates in the particular skills the examination is designed to test. Among the important attributes of an examination are that it should be reproducible and that all candidates should be treated and assessed equally. It is for these reasons that multiple choice questions (MCQ) have been adopted and are increasingly used as one form of objective assessment in medicine.

An objective examination is one in which each candidate answers the same paper under the same conditions, all responses being assessed in exactly the same way, without any subjective bias or influence from examiners. The mark given for every possible response is determined beforehand. In addition to MCQ, objective tests that have been used in medicine include the 'erasive patient management problem' in which a case history is presented and a series of options offered, opposite each of which is an instruction, or additional information concealed from the candidate. Having made his choice, the candidate is able to reveal the item by using one of a variety of techniques to erase the over-print mask. In this way the candidate works through a series of decisions, and marking depends on the appropriate nature of his choices and the number of decisions he has taken in 'managing' the problem presented. The modified essay question (Knox, 1975) is another useful objective technique, and attempts have been made (with varying degrees of success) to conduct clinical examinations that are entirely objective. Most recently, Fleming (1975) has described the missing-link question (MLQ), which is a method of testing candidates' ability to recall and manipulate factual information. This format comprises the insertion of a term which forms a logical link between two other, given, terms. This method seems to discriminate reliably between good and poor candidates.

However, the most familiar objective examination and certainly that most commonly employed is the MCQ paper, which has been used for many years as a reliable measure of knowledge and as a means of accurately discriminating between candidates. The MCQ paper mainly tests recall of factual information and has the unrivalled ability to give an unambiguous and reproducible assessment of knowledge over a wide field. It is, however, now accepted that good MCQ can test more than simple factual recall and a well-prepared paper can test powers of judgement and discrimination as well as the ability to reason. As Lennox (1974) has stated, the intelligent application of well-understood principles and probabilities will often earn better dividends than plain memory work in answering an MCQ test. It must nevertheless be appreciated that different types of examination test different strengths and weaknesses, and it would be unreasonable to expect a conventional MCQ paper to assess adequately all of those qualities that the qualifying undergraduate must possess.

In the earlier days of MCQ, students and teachers often regarded the technique with suspicion, and some still do. Students protested against its impersonal nature (until they appreciated that it was essentially fair) and, justifiably, against the ambiguity of poor questions. Teachers were often uncertain what qualities were in fact being tested and sometimes felt that their roles as assessors were being usurped by the computer. This anxiety was due to a combination of unfamiliarity with the technique, suspicion of a new method of assessment in which the teachers were only involved in the setting of questions and not the assessment of the answers, a high prevalence of poor questions that brought the technique into disrepute in some quarters, and finally the fact that some teachers expected far too much from the MCQ paper and did not realize its limitations. To some extent anxiety about the method persists today (Dudley, 1973), but in general MCQ have been accepted both by students and teachers as an important and valuable means of assessment. Just as acceptance has increased over the years, so the questions used have increased tremendously in 'quality' (with a consequent increase in the reproducibility, discriminating power and validity of the examinations) and methods of analysis of the results have become much more sophisticated, valid and useful. The MCQ has been the subject of many scientific studies that have given valuable information covering the whole field of medical education.

Types of Multiple Choice Question

The simplest form of 'multiple' choice question is the yes/no alternative, e.g.

> Is Edinburgh west of Newcastle?
>
> A. Yes
>
> B. No
>
> (Correct answer: A)

This simply tests factual recall and nothing else; it has no place in medical examinations.

In the UK two basic formats of MCQ are used. Both consist of an initial statement (or stem) followed by a number of possible completions or subsidiary statements (items).

The one-from-five type This asks the student to select a single correct answer from a group of five alternatives. It is important to recognize that in this format what is wanted is not necessarily the *only* possible answer but the 'best' answer of those given and it is wise to reinforce this principle by the wording of the stem. Three examples of the one-from-five type of question are shown below.

> A 46-year-old male patient who is moderately obese is suspected of having Cushing's disease. The *single* observation which would give *most* support to this diagnosis would be:
>
> A. urinary 17-oxosteroid excretion of 80 μmol/24 h (23 mg/24 h)

B. a midnight plasma cortisol of 555 nmol/l (20 μg/100 ml)

C. a blood-pressure of 170/110

D. a diabetic glucose tolerance curve

E. the presence of pink abdominal striae

(Correct answer: B)

The most reliable *single* test that would best support a diagnosis of primary hypothyroidism in a 35-year-old female patient who is taking an oestrogen/progestogen oral contraceptive would be

A. estimation of serum protein bound iodine concentration

B. estimation of serum cholesterol concentration

C. examination of an electrocardiogram

D. examination of the blood for the presence of circulating antibodies to thyroid components

E. estimation of serum TSH concentration

(Correct answer: E)

A man of 68 presents with a sudden episode of severe colicky abdominal pain. Within three days of admission to hospital he becomes jaundiced and develops a high fluctuating pyrexia. The *most likely* diagnosis in this patient is

A. infective hepatitis

B. cirrhosis of the liver

C. a stone impacted in the common bile duct

D. carcinoma of the head of the pancreas

E. an intrahepatic abscess

(Correct answer: C)

The multiple (or grouped) true/false variety The basic format is as for the one-from-five type, but each item is independent of all the others and the candidate has to determine whether each of the items is true or false in its own right. There is no reason why all the items should not be true or why none should be true, and the candidate is allowed to indicate 'don't know' if he wishes. Two examples are given below.

Characteristic features of Cushing's syndrome include

A. generalized obesity (false)

B. hypertension (true)

    C. menorrhagia (false)

    D. proximal muscle weakness (true)

    E. loss of body hair (false)

    F. osteoporosis (true)

Osteitis deformans (Paget's disease of bone)

    A. is more common over the age of 50 than below that age (true)

    B. gives rise to symptoms in the majority of affected patients (false)

    C. is accompanied by elevation of the serum inorganic phosphorus concentration (false)

    D. may be complicated by cardiac failure (true)

    E. responds to treatment with prednisolone (false)

Many variations can be played on this theme. In Newcastle we have found the clinically-based, problem-solving MCQ to be of great value. Here the student is presented with a lengthy stem that describes a clinical problem. Data, in the form of biochemical results, E.C.G.s, X-rays, clinical photographs, photomicrographs etc., are provided to supplement the stem. The items are based on the stem and the data provided. Examples of this type of question are shown in Figs 1.1, 1.2, 1.3 and 1.4. While these cannot replace the conventional clinical examination they do provide an objective type of clinical test and they certainly assess much more than factual recall. Well-prepared questions often discriminate between candidates at a very high level of significance, and this type of question has proved popular with students.

Advantages and disadvantages of one-from-five and multiple true/false. If well prepared, each form of question can yield very good results, although each has some disadvantages. The one-from-five type tests judgement and discrimination to a greater extent than the multiple true/false variety but is more difficult to prepare. All the items in one-from-five must be plausible although one must be more 'correct' than the others and if the examination is to be successful the views of the examiner and the candidates must agree. At the same time the incorrect items (negative distractors) must be such that the correct answer does not stick out like a sore thumb. In addition, the one-from-five format will, in a sixty-question paper, test only sixty items of knowledge — those relating to the stem of the question. The multiple true/false variety runs the risk of increasing the chances that candidates might guess the answers, but these chances have been substantially reduced by offering a 'don't know' option. In many questions of this type the candidate is required to use less judgement than in the one-from-five type, but the extent to which judgement and discrimination are tested largely depends on the care

Figure 1.1 Problem-solving clinical MCQ (Multiple true/false). Emphasis on biochemical data

A 54 year old man was admitted as an emergency with confusion, disorientation, pains in his extremities and dyspnoea a few weeks after an attack of 'flu. He had a past history of meningitis at 28 which left him with a cauda equina lesion and a hypotonic bladder. Following bladder neck resection he had become incontinent and he wore a portable urinal. He had suffered recurrent urinary infections and was being followed in the out-patient clinic on account of stable chronic renal failure with a typical plasma urea of about 100 mg/100 ml.

On admission he had deep respirations of 24/min. There were a few crepitations at the lung bases but chest x-ray was normal. There was impaired sensation in both hands and the sensory deficit in his lower limbs was more extensive than at previous out-patient visits.

Initial investigation showed plasma urea 308 mg/100 ml, creatinine 15·2 mg/100 ml, Na 141 mEq/L, K 4·5 mEq/L, Cl 111 mEq/L, HCO_3 4 mEq/L, blood pH 7·06, $PaCO_2$ 16, base deficit greater than 22 mEq/L, buffer base 20 mEq/L, Standard Bicarb. 6 mEq/L, Serum Ca. 5·3 mg/l00 ml, PO_4, 12·3 mg/100 ml, total proteins 6·7 mg/100 ml, A1b. 4·0 g/100 ml.

- − A His blood acid-base changes could be explained by repeated vomiting over the three days before admission
- − B There is biochemical evidence of serious pulmonary pathology interfering with gaseous diffusion
- + C Intravenous calcium gluconate or chloride should be given before his acid base derangement is corrected
- − D His plasma urea is very high in relationship to his plasma creatinine indicating that he has been eating a high protein diet
- − E The sensory changes in his hands are best explained by a late effect of his meningitis causing scarring around the cervical nerve roots
- + F He will probably require diuretics and/or dialysis to prevent fluid overload while his metabolic state is being corrected

with which the questions are set and phrased. In a sixty-question paper, three hundred different items of knowledge can be tested. Depending on the stems, these may, within a single question, be more or less closely related. Thus in the same question one can ask about aetiology, diagnosis and management of a disease and one need not confine oneself to a single aspect of the condition. On the other hand, a question may deal with one aspect in depth. The multiple true/false format is much more flexible and permissive than the one-from-five variety. Both of the question formats can be very useful indeed, but I have a preference for the multiple true/false type. This is influenced by the feeling that more 'mileage' can be got out of the multiple true/false question and the fact that a really convincing one-from-five question is much more difficult to set. A poorly set one-from-five means that five items are wasted; a poorly set multiple true/false (unless quite catastrophic) may only be pulled down by one or two items, which can, on revision of a question, be replaced. Three important points must be made. The first is that multiple choice questions of either variety are not easy to set and great care must be taken if the question is to be a good and valid test of knowledge and judgement, and a useful discriminator. The second point is that while each type of question has value the types can not readily be mixed in the same paper since each requires a different method of scoring. Thirdly, the two-question forms are not readily interchangeable. For one thing, the wording of the stem of a one-from-five will almost certainly need altering to fit the multiple true/false format. For another, the answer key will probably need to be altered, usually converting a good one-from-five to an inferior multiple true/false. A question conceived as a one-from-five will, if marked as a multiple true/false, yield a totally inappropriate score. Similarly, although a multiple true/false question may only contain one true item, this does *not* mean that it can be used as a one-from-five question. The whole concept of the two forms is different — the key feature of one-from-five is that *all* of the items are plausible and up to a point correct — one is *more* correct than the others and the candidate is asked to select this item.

Other Complex Variants

There are other types of MCQ which are used much less in the UK than in the USA. These have been described in detail by Hubbard and Clemans (1961) and include the *multiple completion type* in which a stem is followed by a series of numbered statements and the candidate is asked (for instance) to select (a) if all statements are correct, (b) if none are correct, (c) if statements 1 and 2 are correct, (d) if 1, 2 and 3 are correct and (e) if 2 and 4 are correct. A second complex variant is the *relationship analysis type*. Here the candidate is presented with a statement containing a fact and a reason and asked (for example) to select (a) if both fact and reason are true and related as to cause and effect, (b) if both are true but no causal relation is present, (c) if the

Figure 1.2 Problem-solving clinical MCQ (Multiple true/false). Various data given

A man of 45 was referred to the outpatient department with a three year history of weight gain of 40 Kg (88 lbs.) up to his present level of 115 Kg (254 lbs.), tiredness, husky voice, and puffiness of the face and lower legs. There was no past history of note. He was a sluggish, obese man with a dry cool skin. The pulse was 64 per minute, and the blood pressure 140/80. There was some pitting oedema of the feet and shins. His PBI was 1·4 micrograms per 100 ml, serum cholesterol 445 mg/100 ml, serum proteins total 8·1 G./100 ml (albumin 3·5 G., globulin 4·6 G.), Serum flocculations: Zinc sulphate 10, Thymol turbidity 7, Thymol flocculation + + + . There was slight proteinuria (less than 1 G./24 hours), but no significant urinary deposit. Blood urea 35 mg/100 ml, electrolytes normal. Haemoglobin 13·9 G./100 ml. Anti-thyroglobulin antibodies positive to a titre of 1 in 2,000,000. Skull x-ray normal. Two electrocardiograms (one taken before treatment and the other six months after treatment had been started) are shown. A photograph taken when he was first seen is also shown.

− A The difference between the two electrocardiograms is due to evolution of a cardiac infarction
+ B It would be expected that the relaxation phase of the ankle jerk will be prolonged
− C A thyrotropin stimulation test is strongly indicated
− D The serum protein and flocculation results indicate that hepatic cirrhosis should be suspected, since they cannot be explained on the basis of the data given
− E A history of pernicious anaemia in his mother would be purely fortuitous
− F Violaceous thickened areas of skin over the shins are a typical finding in this condition

Pre Rx

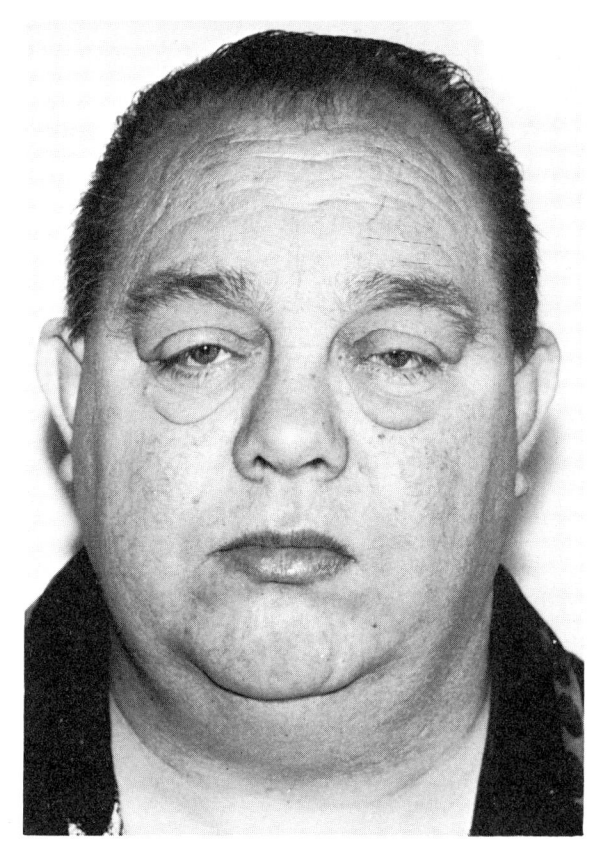

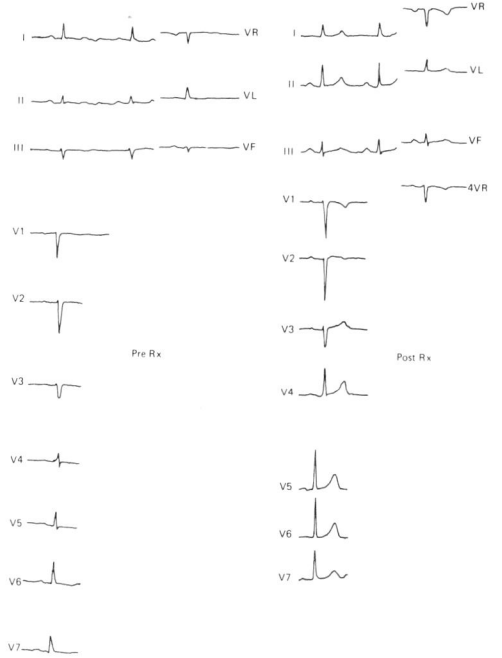

Post Rx

9

Figure 1.3 Problem-solving clinical MCQ (Multiple true/false). X-ray and brief history

A 65 year old farmer gives a four year history of increasing pain, stiffness and deformity in the left hip, with a limp for six months. Among the physical signs elicited is a severe flexion-adduction contracture of the left hip. An X-ray of the left hip joint is shown. This man

- − A will have an increase in the apparent length of the left leg
- − B should be treated in the first instance with oral and intra-articular cortico-steroids
- + C should be advised to use a walking stick in the right hand
- + D will have a positive Thomas's test on the left
- − E will be found to have more than 25,000 white blood cells per cubic millimetre in synovial fluid aspirated from the left hip joint

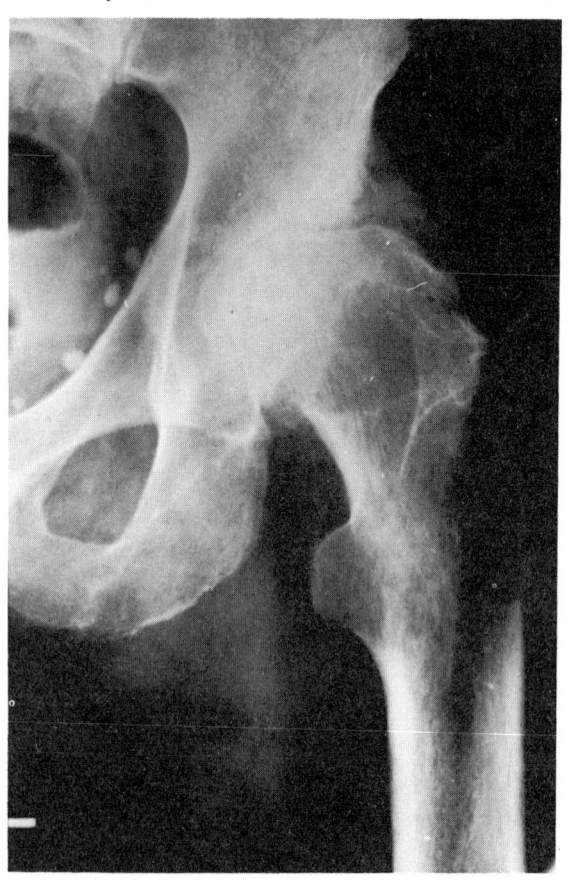

fact is true but not the cause, (d) if the cause is true but not the fact
and (e) if neither is true. These are variants on the multiple true/false
theme and some even more complex examples have been published and
used. These formats have been widely adopted in the USA and Canada

Figure 1.4 Problem-solving clinical MCQ (Multiple true/false). Clinical
and other data

A 23 year old woman is now at the 38th week of pregnancy. She had an uneventful pregnancy until the 35th week when she was noticed to have a blood pressure of 130/90 and the fundal height was recorded as 30 cm. She was admitted to hospital and since then her blood pressure has remained at that level in spite of sedation with diazepam 5 mg. twice a day. Serial urinary total oestrogens have been performed as well as serial fundal height estimations [**8a**]. Gestational amniocentesis was performed at 37 weeks and the result stated that "the gestational age is compatible with the dates". Labour was induced at 10.00 hours today by artificial rupture of the membranes and Syntocinon delivered through the Cardiff pump system. At 14.00 hours the uterus was contracting 1:3 and she was becoming distressed. Her B.P. was 140/100. A vaginal examination was performed and the cervix was found to be 4 cm. dilated. A fetal scalp electrode and intra uterine pressure tube were introduced and connected to the cardiotocograph. The appearances of the trace are shown [**8b**].

+ A   The serial steroid and uterine measurements [**8a**] suggest that the fetus is probably suffering from intra uterine growth retardation
− B   The cardiotocograph tracing [**8b**] suggests that the fetus is suffering from acute hypoxia
+ C   An epidural anaesthetic is indicated at this stage
− D   She should be delivered by Caesarean section within the next hour
− E   There is a high risk that this infant will develop respiratory distress syndrome

TOTAL OESTROGEN (μg/24 hrs)   FUNDAL HEIGHT (cms)

8a Closed circles: normal values; open circles: patient's results

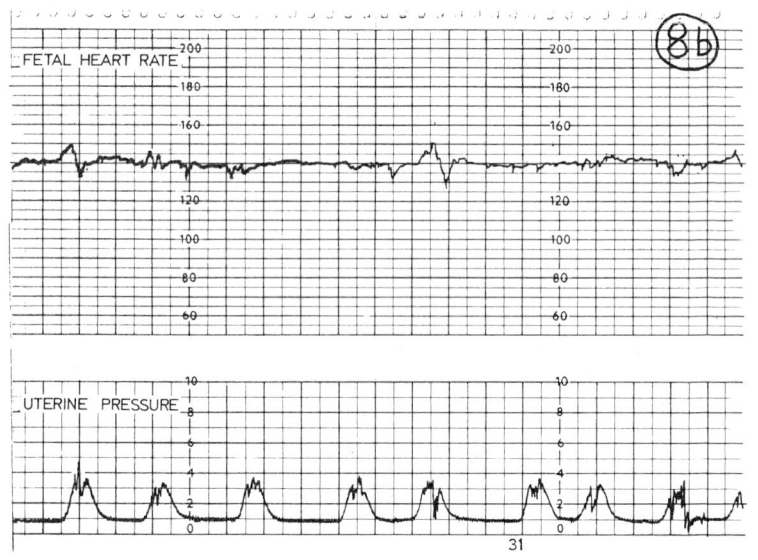

Figure 1.4 (continued)

but the general view is that they are not usually suitable for use in the United Kingdom. Very often these complex types of MCQ have evolved more as a result of constraints imposed by the computer program used to mark them than because of any inherent theoretical educational advantage they may have — the two varieties described above attempt to introduce a multiple true/false format to questions marked by a one-from-five program. Their complexity confuses those who meet them for the first time, and they are as much a test of intelligence and command of the English language as of medical knowledge; although this may not always be a bad thing, the mental gymnastics required to decide simply what the question is trying to ask are often formidable. Since these formats do not conform to the aims of MCQ usually laid down in the UK, nothing more will be said about them.

In Newcastle the multiple true/false format has been used for almost twenty years and a great deal of experience has been obtained during this time. This type is widely favoured in the UK and is probably used more often overall than the one-from-five variety. Certainly the multiple true/false format is used in many medical schools and by the great majority of postgraduate examining bodies. Since the marking program described later has been designed for this type of question, with progressive refinement and improvement over the years, it is mainly this type that will be discussed in this book — all of the examples given later are of this form. Nevertheless, many of the statements made apply equally well to both the multiple true/false and the one-from-five varieties and where a statement does not apply to the latter format this will be made clear.

CHAPTER TWO

Setting of Multiple Choice Questions

THE KEYS TO the successful writing of MCQ are precision and clarity. A poorly set MCQ is valueless as a means of assessment — indeed, the results it produces may be frankly misleading. Such MCQ only serve to bring the technique into disrepute and increase candidates' and examiners' suspicions of the method. This chapter outlines some of the common faults and is intended mainly for examiners, although it is hoped that it will also be of help to candidates and serve to reassure them.

The aim of MCQ examiners is to set a paper that tests the candidates' knowledge, powers of judgement and of discrimination. We do not attempt to set an intelligence test — there are much better ways of assessing intelligence (and of a knowledge of the English language and its vagaries) than asking a candidate to unravel the meaning of a complex and wordy question. The wording of the questions, therefore, should be kept as simple as possible so that the candidate is left in no doubt as to what he is required to do and is not inconvenienced and handicapped by having to interpret the question as well as give the answers. The wording of each stem and each item must therefore be unambiguous.

In his book, *The Complete Plain Words* (revised by Sir Bruce Fraser, 1973) Sir Ernest Gowers gave the following three general rules for the clear and correct use of English:

> 'Use no more words than are necessary to express your meaning, for if you use more you are likely to obscure it and to tire your reader. In particular, do not use superfluous adjectives and adverbs and do not use roundabout phrases where single words would serve.
>
> Use familiar words rather than the far-fetched, if they express your meaning equally well, for the familiar are more likely to be readily understood.
>
> Use words with a precise meaning rather than those that are vague, for they will obviously serve better to make your meaning clear; and in particular, prefer concrete words to abstract, for they are more likely to have a precise meaning.'

The person who sets MCQ will not go far wrong if he attempts to follow these rules. A question that is vague and ambiguous will not discriminate well between candidates, since they will all be puzzled by its wording. Different candidates will interpret the question in different ways and many will finally guess. These principles apply equally to the multiple true/false and to the one-from-five formats. However, it was pointed out in the first chapter that these two types ask different things of the candidate — the multiple true/false type asks him to regard each item as independent of all the others and to answer whether each is a true or false statement. The one-from-five variety asks the candidate to select the 'best' answer out of those alternatives given. Because of this, the wording of the stem will differ in the two types, and some methods and procedures commonly used in the one-from-five form will be unacceptable for the multiple true/false. The two types are therefore dealt with separately in the discussion that follows.

The Setting of Multiple True/False Questions

Topics and content   Questions can be set which relate to every medical discipline but while ideas for question themes are obviously important, the ability to compose a precisely worded question on a particular topic is equally important. All teachers and examiners involved should be encouraged to submit questions, since this broadens the field and increases the variety of topics. Setters of questions should be given some elementary advice on the form which their submissions should take and of the basic traps they should avoid. At the same time all questions submitted are best reviewed and edited by an individual or a small group experienced in the wording of questions. In the case of courses or departments that define the objectives of their teaching, the content of the paper will clearly be influenced, although the final presentation of the questions is still of critical importance.

A good MCQ examination assesses the medical knowledge of candidates and discriminates between them on this basis. It is therefore important that the questions should be pitched at the right level: there is little point in setting a question that is so difficult that nobody can answer it correctly. Similarly, the question that is so easy that all get it right is of no discriminatory value. Questions that all candidates *are* expected to get right are of some value in certain types of examination designed to test whether the objectives of a course of study have been achieved and to ensure that some basic and important aspects of medicine are understood. There would be justifiable concern if students, after a course of endocrinology lectures, demonstrated a total lack of knowledge in answering a question dealing with basic clinical aspects of thyrotoxicosis or if, after a course on respiratory disease, a majority indicated that patients in respiratory failure should be treated with morphine. Nevertheless, it must be clearly understood that questions used for these purposes as well as those that are too difficult will not discriminate between good and weak candidates since all will be either 'good' or 'weak'. No paper should be set by one person alone, although an individual may be responsible for editing the questions submitted. If we are to be realistic we should confine questions to the more important aspects of medical knowledge, although this depends on the aims of a particular examination. Certainly personal views and prejudices which are not part of the generally accepted body of medical knowledge should be avoided. Questions should only ask for information that the candidate should be expected to know or to deduce without consulting a reference source. Drug dosages, limits of normal values and other numerical data should be included only if they deal with data that are within the daily working knowledge of the candidate, whether he is an undergraduate or a postgraduate.

Wording In the multiple true/false format the candidate is presented with an initial statement or stem followed by a number of completions or items identified by letters. He is asked to indicate whether he considers each item to be true or false and is allowed to indicate 'don't know' where appropriate. Each item is independent and is given equal weighting. The stem and the items may together form a statement, as in the examples shown below:

Impetigo

A. can complicate pediculosis capitis (true)

Characteristic features of Addisonian pernicious anaemia include

A. an increased liability to neurological complications if treated with folic acid alone (true)

B. duodenal ulcer (false)

Alternatively each item may be a statement complete in itself:

The following statements are correct:

A. Return of gastric hydrochloric acid secretion after successful treatment with vitamin B_{12} is a characteristic feature of Addisonian pernicious anaemia (false)

Every possible care must be taken to avoid ambiguity, both in the stem and in the items. It must be realized that the better student may see an ambiguous point in an item which might be less obvious to the plodder. Such a question might possibly handicap the better student and is therefore unsuitable. Stems should be phrased so that the words 'true' or 'false' are logical and grammatical answers, e.g., *The following statements are correct* – not *Which of the following statements are correct?* One must avoid indicating in the stem how many items should be marked 'true', e.g., *The most likely diagnosis is; The three commonest causes of ... are ....*

In both stem and items absolute terms such as *always*, *never*, etc., should be avoided since the astute candidate will realize that, except in a tiny fraction of examples, the answer must be false. Such terms are sometimes permissible if the correct answer is 'true', although it is unlikely that this will occur very often. If the terms *are* to be used in MCQ, they must be taken to imply 'without any exceptions'. Vague words such as *often, commonly, rare, urgently, emergency, routine, sometimes, frequently,* etc., should, if possible, be avoided (Gibson, 1969; Castle, 1976) and it is the use of words such as these that has been responsible for more criticism of MCQ than any other fault. How often is often? How common is common? How urgent is urgent? Such imprecise words may sometimes 'work' if the correct answer is unequivocally 'false', but they should not be used in items that are 'true' and it is best to avoid them altogether if possible. By doing this the wording of questions may become stereotyped, but better this than that there should be any uncertainty in the minds of candidates. Terms that give an exact percentage frequency (*25% of cases*) are best avoided since they imply that 24% or 26% may be wrong answers and medicine is never as precise as this. Such items might be permissible as false items if the figure given is so wrong as to avoid any possibility of argument. This, however, is likely to produce an item which is far too easy. Phrases such as *less than 25%, more than 80%* are more acceptable, as are proportions, such as *more than two thirds, less than a quarter,* provided that the terms are used with care and there is no possibility that the candidate might be misled. The term *the majority* is acceptable; it should be taken to mean 'at least 50%'. The phrase *is associated with* should not be used. Just about anything can be 'associated' with anything. However, qualification of this phrase is acceptable: . . . *is significantly associated with . . ., . . . typically associated with . . ., . . . recognized association.*

These vague words and phrases have led to the evolution of a number of standard terms used in the wording of stems. These include *recognized, characteristic* and *typical.* Thus, *recognized complications of . . . include, characteristic features of . . . include, the following features are typical of . . ..* Even here problems may arise in theory since the dictionary definitions of these words tend to lack precision and clarity. However, problems rarely arise in practice and candidates seem able to interpret without difficulty questions that use these terms.

A *characteristic feature* (or *complication, change, finding*) is not necessarily one that 'characterizes' the disease in that it occurs in *that* disease (even though it may only be seen in 1% of patients) and in *no* other but is one which occurs so often as, usually, to be of some diagnostic significance and, if it were not present, might lead to doubt being cast on the diagnosis. Examples of this might be:

Characteristic features of secondary syphilis include

A. positive serological tests for syphilis (true)

Characteristic changes of diabetic retinopathy include

A. retinal microaneurysms (true)

Characteristic features of osteomalacia due to a deficient intake of vitamin D include

A. a lower than normal serum inorganic phosphorus concentration (true)

A *recognized feature* (or *complication*, etc.) is one that, although it may not 'characterize' a disease, has been reported and that is a fact a candidate would reasonably be expected to know. Thus all 'characteristic' features are 'recognized' but many 'recognized' features could not be described as 'characteristic':

Recognized complications of primary hyperparathyroidism include

A. peptic ulceration (true)

This association is certainly 'well-recognized' but would not be regarded as 'characteristic' (although hypercalcaemia would).

Recognized unwanted effects of metformin include

A. malabsorption of vitamin B_{12} (true)

B. peripheral neuropathy (false)

The following statements are correct:

A. Duodenal ulcer is a recognized association of Addisonian pernicious anaemia (false)

B. Primary amenorrhoea is a recognized feature of Turner's syndrome (true)

In B the word 'recognized' could equally well, in this case, be 'characteristic'.

The term *typical* is more or less synonymous with *characteristic*. A *typical* feature is one that one would expect to be present.

Pathognomonic and *specific* indicate features that occur in the disease named and in no other.

It can be argued that by introducing terms such as *recognized* and *characteristic* in place of *often* and *commonly* the setter of multiple choice questions has replaced one set of imprecise terms by another. In fact, experience of multiple choice questions indicates that the former terms are not misinterpreted by candidates and the choice of which to use causes more anxiety to the setter, who should simply strive for the greatest accuracy and clarity. Provided that questions are set with care and that the terms are used in the right context, *recognized*, *characteristic* and *typical* do not puzzle candidates and are much less ambiguous and misleading than *common*, etc. In any case, even if a stem or item does cause confusion, the candidate need not be penalized since this can be compensated for in the marking process (see Chapter 4).

The wording of MCQ is best illustrated by an example. Let us suppose that the examiner wishes to ask a question about thyroid antibodies and myxoedema. How should the item be worded?

1. Patients with myxoedema sometimes have positive thyroid antibodies.
   NO They may *sometimes* have ingrowing toenails; patients with ingrowing toe-nails *sometimes* have positive thyroid antibodies. There is no implicit causal relationship. A sloppy way of wording the item (although one must admit that it is so permissive as to avoid misinterpretation in this case — all right for a 'true' but certainly not for a 'false').

2. Patients with myxoedema often (commonly) have positive thyroid antibodies.
   NO Just as sloppy and again too permissive. How often? How common? How positive? Which antibodies?

3. 99% of patients with myxoedema have positive antibodies.
   NO Too wrong, just as 2%, and the absolute terms *always* and *never* would be too obviously wrong.

4. More than half of patients with myxoedema have positive thyroid antibodies.
   NO Better, but does myxoedema mean primary thyroid failure? What type of antibody? The statement would be correct for the complement fixation or tanned red cell tests but not for precipitin tests.

5. Circulating antibodies to thyroglobulin are a recognized feature of primary hypothyroidism.
   YES The only safe and foolproof way of testing this item of knowledge. Cannot be misinterpreted. (*NB:* Characteristic is not an appropriate term here but *would be* if the condition was Hashimoto's thyroiditis. Apologies for the subtlety, but I hope readers will now get the point).

Precision In an attempt to achieve brevity, most of us are at times rather imprecise in our speech. Thus we talk about 'lung cancer' rather than specifying 'primary bronchial carcinoma', 'leukaemia' instead of specifying the type and 'myxoedema' without qualifying whether this is due to primary thyroid failure or secondary to hypopituitarism. Sometimes 'diabetes' will be referred to without defining whether this is diabetes mellitus or diabetes insipidus. In most cases the context makes our intentions clear, but this may not always be so in MCQ, where great precision is needed. When 'treatment' is referred to, it may sometimes be necessary to qualify this by adjectives such as 'successful', 'effective', 'adequate' or 'appropriate' or the dosage of a drug that is used may even need to be given. When drugs are mentioned they should always be printed as the generic name with (if thought appropriate) the proprietary name in brackets afterwards. If the terms 'low dosage' or 'high dosage' are mentioned, they should always be clarified by actually giving the dose. It may sometimes be necessary to add the phrase '... in the United Kingdom' to avoid any possibility of confusion. Eponymous names for diseases should be used with caution and should preferably be associated with an alternative name, e.g., Down's syndrome (mongolism); juvenile rheumatoid arthritis (Still's disease) unless no suitable alternative term is available and the eponymous term is quite unambiguous, e.g., Crohn's disease; Henoch-Schönlein syndrome; Huntington's chorea.

There are many such examples and the setter of MCQ must ask himself: 'bearing in mind the wording I have used, could the answers I regard as being correct become incorrect or doubtful in *any* other circumstances that the wording does not exclude? Have I been specific enough to make my meaning absolutely clear to the candidate?'

Mutually exclusive items None of the items given should be mutually exclusive, interdependent or interrelated, i.e., the answer to one item should not automatically give, imply or even influence the answer to another:

A blood glucose of 1·1 mmol/l (20 mg per dl) indicates

A. hypoglycaemia

B. hyperglycaemia

Propranolol causes

A. bronchial constriction

B. bronchial dilatation

The reason for avoiding items like this is that in the marking system equal weighting is given for correct 'false' answers as well as for correct 'true' answers. In the examples given above the candidate would, by knowing only one item of information, score two marks. Not all examples of mutually exclusive items are as gross as those given above, and great care must be taken in setting questions that one item does not give any clue to the answer of another. It is a useful exercise to scrutinize each item critically with this in mind after a question is set. The question to ask is 'if item A is correct (or incorrect) does *any* other item then automatically become incorrect (or correct)?' Care must be taken to avoid asking the same question in different ways in two separate items.

Not all items that are direct opposites are automatically mutually exclusive; both might sometimes be correct:

Juvenile hypothyroidism may be causally related to

    A. a lower than normal thyroidal uptake of radioactive iodine (true)

    B. a higher than normal thyroidal uptake of radioactive iodine (true)

Negatives Stem formats that superficially look alike but that differ in sense must be avoided, and this is particularly true of negatives. It is very easy for the candidate who is under stress to miss the negative in an otherwise standard form of words and therefore to misinterpret the question. Negatives in the stem and the items are best avoided: *the following are not recognized features of . . ..* These tricks only serve to confuse the candidate and add nothing to the value of the question. Double negatives (*not uncommon, not unlikely that, not unexpected*) should not be used. As well as confusing the harassed British candidate their subtle nuances may not be understood by the candidate whose native tongue is other than English.

Double-barrelled items Items which contain two 'bits' of knowledge are best avoided, even when both phrases are correct (or incorrect). An example is:

    Propranolol causes

    A. bradycardia and hypotension (true)

These actions would best be tested in two separate items. Such double-barrelled items must never be used when one phrase is correct and one incorrect:

    Propranolol causes

    A. bradycardia and hypertension

    In a grossly obese patient with maturity-onset diabetes treatment should be with

    A. a weight-reducing diet (true) and a sulphonylurea (false)

Such errors of setting may occur in a subtle way:

    A patient with myxoedema coma

    A. should be treated with large doses (false) of tri-iodothyronine (true), given intravenously (contentious).

The rule should always be: one item, one fact.

A word of warning When setting a question, the first item or two you write down will almost certainly be true, and you will then start to search for false statements for the later items. It is surprising how consistent this pattern of item arrangement seems to be and the pattern can be detected by the best candidates. For this reason it is best to 'scramble' the items or arrange them at random once you have decided on them.

Special Considerations for One-from-Five Questions

Much of what has been said in the preceding sections applies to the setting of one-from-five questions as well as multiple true/false, but there are also a number of important differences. Precise, clear and specific wording is still very important but the basic principle of the one-from-five question is that only one item is correct and that the others are incorrect. This principle will often be apparent in the wording of the stems: *which one of the following . . .?* The setting of stems requires careful thought since they must be worded with complete precision to avoid two answers being equally 'correct' while at the same time making it possible to devise convincing negatives that may not sometimes be right. Negatives in the stem are more acceptable than in the multiple true/false variety but should be emphasized when they occur, if necessary by underlining. Absolute terms are sometimes used since *never*, although strictly false, may still be the nearest to truth of the responses given. A number of variant formats are sometimes used. These include the 'order finding' type of question, where five items are presented and the candidates are asked which item would occupy a particular place if they were put in the proper order. These variants are fully reviewed by Lennox (1974) in his booklet on the setting and evaluation of this type of question, but many of these alternative forms all introduce possible new hazards.

Just as there is sometimes bias in the order in which items are placed in multiple true/false questions, similar bias may be seen in the one-from-five type of question where there is often a natural reluctance to put the correct answer first, and randomization of the items is recommended. Other irrelevant clues that may point to the correct answer should be avoided; they include the correct item that is longer and more precise than the distractors, the use of common elements in the stem and the correct item and inadvertent grammatical clues.

Setting an MCQ Paper

Although the wider the breadth of opinion available to comment on a potential MCQ paper the better, it has many advantages if a single individual, with some experience in the technique, is responsible for the preliminary stages in the setting procedure. This person will in effect be the secretary of the examining body and will usually be responsible for maintaining the question bank, for seeing that it remains adequately stocked and for obtaining new questions. He will compile the paper for approval by the examiners and will include in it a series of new questions (which he may or may not edit first), some questions that have been used previously and revised and some 'marker' questions (see Chapter 5) that are to be used again in an unaltered form. The preliminary paper may be circulated by the secretary to the examiners in advance of the setting meeting, together with brief comments on the questions, or may only be seen by the examiners for the first time at the meeting. The secretary will attempt to select a balanced series of questions that cover, according to the objectives and scope of the examination, the whole field to be tested.

The examiners will scrutinize each question, paying particular attention to relevance, degree of difficulty and clarity. Some poor or ambiguous questions will be discarded, others will have changes made to either the stem or to the items or both (sometimes these may only involve minor syntactical alterations), and some questions will be accepted as they stand. Marker questions should not be altered unless there is some compelling reason to do so, otherwise they lose their status as markers. It is advisable for the secretary to have some questions in reserve at the meeting, or to have easy and immediate access to such questions, to replace any that the examiners have discarded and to maintain the desired balance.

The answer key must be carefully checked by the secretary during his preliminary compilation, at the examiners' meeting and again when the paper is prepared in its final form for submission to the printers. Printers' proofs should, if possible be checked by more than one person. The answer key and the numbered candidate list together with any special requests for group sorting should be sent to the computing laboratory (if the examination is to be computer marked) as far in advance of the examination as possible.

CHAPTER THREE

Candidate Responses—Lector and Opscan Sheets

Multiple true/false questions

The candidate must have some means of indicating his answers to the questions, his responses must be 'read' and recorded accurately and they must be converted to a format suitable for scoring and analysis. It is of course possible to hand-mark answer sheets of the multiple true/false type, but this is tedious and, unless carefully undertaken, prone to error. Hand-marked answer sheets simply require the candidate to insert ticks (or true/false responses) on a grid (item letters along the top and question numbers down the side), to ring letters, or even to record his responses adjacent to the items on the question paper. However, although accurate candidate scores can be obtained by this means (see Chapter 4), it is almost impossible to analyse the questions statistically and to assess their discriminatory power in more than a crude way. Printed response sheets and computer marking are therefore used for the great majority of undergraduate and postgraduate examinations where more than a handful of candidates are being assessed.

Like many other aspects of MCQ, candidates' response sheets have gradually changed over the years as new and better techniques of marking have evolved. Such changes have sometimes been associated with alterations to the computer programs used to score the answer sheet — there are several such programs (Hubbard, 1971; Buckley-Sharp and Harris, 1971) and even more response sheets. Those that will be described in this chapter have been used by the University of Newcastle upon Tyne Computing Laboratory for the marking of all the MCQ examinations of the multiple true/false type processed by the Newcastle computer since the early 1960s.

In the earliest MCQ format the candidate was simply required to make an independent 'yes/no' decision on each item. The scoring system required that each question should contain at least one correct and at least one incorrect item. No provision was made for the indication of uncertainty so that failure to select an item as correct was treated as a definite decision that it was incorrect. The candidate was asked to indicate those items he considered correct by ringing the corresponding letters on an answer sheet attached to the question book. Each set of answers, identified by the candidate's number and name, was transferred to eight-hole punched paper tape, verified and fed into the computer. In the early days this process was carried out by punch operators (*Phase one*). Each question was of the standard multiple true/false format referred to in the first chapter and comprised anything from four to nine items (Owen *et al.*, 1967).

In the *second Phase* beginning in 1968, the same basic procedure was still used but the response sheets were read automatically. The candidate was asked to indicate his responses by marking an answer sheet in pencil in the box corresponding to each item. As before, a mark was taken to indicate that the candidate thought the answer was correct; likewise the absence of a mark was regarded as a decision that the candidate felt the answer was incorrect since no provision was made on the response sheet for the indication 'don't know'. A candidate's response could be cancelled by shading in the lower half of the item response box but no alternative response could then be inserted, nor could the original response be reinstated. The candidate's responses were 'read' and transferred by the document-reading machine (the English Electric Lector) to punched paper tape which was then used as input for the computer (English Electric KDF 9). As in *Phase one*, the scoring system gave credit for correctly unselected negative items as well as for correctly selected positive ones, and incorrect selections resulted in loss of marks. This scoring system is described in more detail in Chapter 4, but a major criticism was that the weighting of individual items corresponded to the number of items of the same sign within the question; thus the candidate's score on each item depended not only on his knowledge but also on the number of positive and negative items in the question. After several years it was clear that there were other unsatisfactory features in this system. The most important of these was the limitation of the candidates' choice in each item to either true or false. Very often the absence of a mark indicated that the candidate did not know, and not that he felt that the item was incorrect. Analysis of question performance very often showed a high percentage of 'correct' (i.e. letters not ringed or boxes unmarked) responses to an item for which the key was 'false'. Some of these 'correct' responses came from well-informed candidates who knew that the item *was* 'false' but an unknown number must have come from those who simply did not know. The latter candidates did in fact benefit from this scoring system — the 'hidden bonus'. Furthermore, it seemed undesirable to force the candidate to guess if the item dealt with an area of knowledge with which he was quite unfamiliar. The response sheets were therefore redesigned in 1970 so that the candidate was required to make a positive choice of either 'true' *or* 'false' for each item by marking the appropriate box on the answer sheet (LECTOR SHEET) (*Phase three*) (Fig. 3.1). By failing to mark either box he tacitly admitted his ignorance of that item. The number of items in a question was limited to five or six and candidates were required to draw a firm bold pencil line across the centre of the box they wished to select. A selection could be cancelled by shading in completely the lower half of

Figure 3.1 Lector Sheet (Phase three)

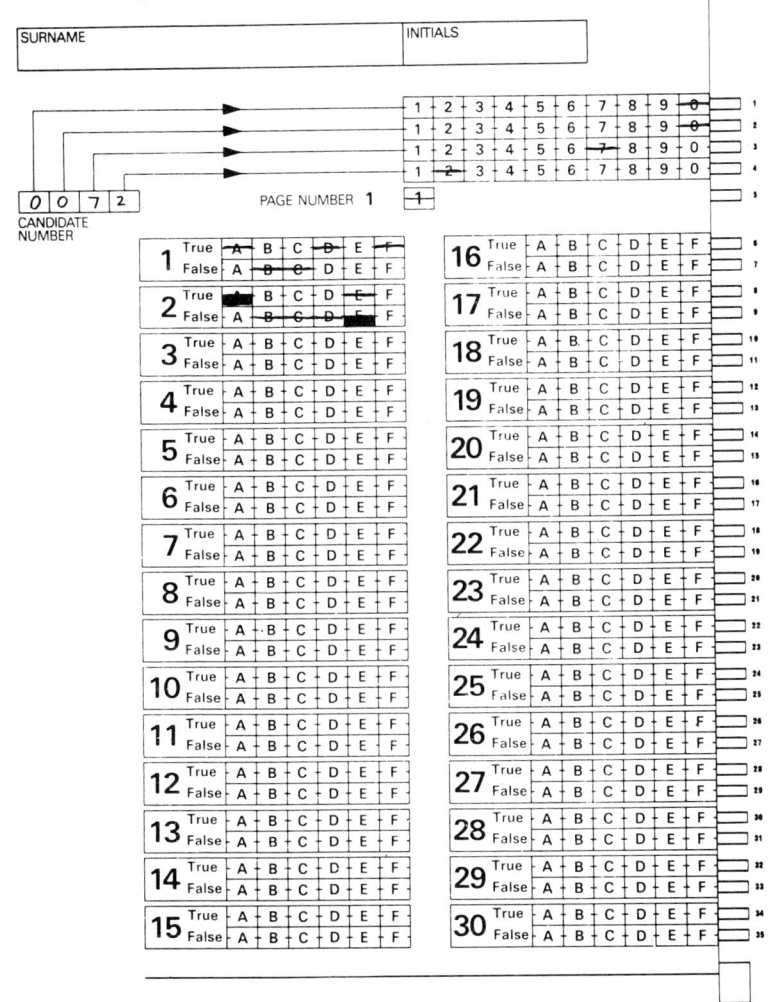

the box, and the candidate was then at liberty to select the alternative response for that item or to leave it blank, indicating 'don't know'. In each case the shaded box was ignored when the paper was marked. There was no restriction on the number of true and false items, and it was possible for all the items in a question to be true or all to be false. The change resulted in an alteration to the marking system, which had the advantage that the weighting of items previously referred to was removed, and each item within a question was scored equally. In the new marking system one mark (+1) was given for each item correctly answered, whether positive or negative. One mark (−1) was deducted for each incorrectly answered item. No marks were given for any item omitted by the candidate or when the candidate marked an item as both true and false. The mark for a single question was obtained by dividing the score for that question by the number of items in the question. This gave a maximum mark of +1 and a minimum mark of −1 for each question. Some 'weighting' still occurred, since a correct response in a five-item question scored 0·2 whereas in a six-item question a correct response scored 0·167. As before, the response sheets (Lector sheets) were marked automatically by the English Electric Lector system and candidate responses were transferred to paper tape for processing by the computer (IBM 360/67).

    The two marking systems have been compared (Fleming *et al.*, 1974). A number of questions set in Part I of the MRCP and MRCP (UK) examinations which had been marked under the old scoring system (*Phase two*) and repeated in later Part I MRCP (UK) examinations which were marked using the new (*Phase three*) scoring system (true/false/don't know) were compared. The two values of the mean scores for these questions gave a very high correlation coefficient. A direct comparison of the mean scores for these questions showed no significant differences for the majority. In a third of the questions the mean score with the original system was significantly greater than that with the new. Correlation coefficients (coefficients of discrimination) for the questions (see Chapter 5) were nearly all higher when the new system was used (Fleming *et al.*, 1974). In summary, therefore, when the new marking system (*Phase three*) was employed, questions tended to have a slightly lower mean score and their discriminatory power was more clearly revealed. The reason for this became apparent when individual items rather than whole questions were compared. In the majority of positive items the 'percentage of candidates correct' was not significantly different whichever system of scoring was used. However, a very different pattern was seen for the negative items of which a large majority had a lower 'percentage candidates correct' when the *Phase three* scoring system was used. It appears that in the old *Phase two* system candidates, by failing to mark an item of which they were uncertain, had in effect correctly indicated it as negative (wrong) and obtained credit for knowledge they did not possess. With the introduction of the 'don't know' option the true extent of the candidates' knowledge and of the discriminatory power of some negative items became apparent. The inflated scores obtained with *Phase two* response sheets when the correct answer to a question was 'false', and candidates gained marks by not marking the item, have been confirmed by Sanderson (1973). Response sheets with facility for indicating 'true/false/don't know' overcame this difficulty but have introduced a new and variable factor into the results which has been studied by Sanderson (1973). Its influence in allowing the candidate to withdraw from answering a question has tended to reduce candidates' scores; this effect is more marked in abler candidates. The factor may well be related to the personalities of those taking the examination and the degree of caution they exercise. Harden *et al.* (1976) have suggested that the 'don't know' option in MCQ papers favours the bold and test-wise student; on the other hand, as mentioned above, the right/wrong response sheet without the 'don't know' option may, in certain circumstances, favour the cautious candidate who is more inclined to avoid making a selection. On balance, the true/false/don't know format seems in practice to be more satisfactory for general use in the 'true' examination situation — some relevant studies have been conducted in an artificial situation. Nevertheless, it would be interesting to determine whether those candidates who are familiar with MCQ react differently (and, I suspect, perform better) than those who have less experience of the technique.

True/false/don't know Lector sheets were used between 1970 and 1975 for all MCQ examinations marked by the Newcastle computer. In 1975 a new document reader (Opscan 17—Interscan Data Systems (UK) Ltd) and a new response sheet, the Opscan sheet (Fig. 3.2), were introduced — *Phase four*. These, like the Lector sheets, are read automatically but the machine is 'on-line' and the output is transferred direct to a small computer where the data are stored on magnetic tape or on disks before being transferred to the main computer (IBM 370/168) for scoring.

Candidates retain the choice of indicating 'true', 'false' or 'don't know' and the marking system is unaltered (see Chapter 4). However, the automatic marking of response sheets using the Opscan system is much more rapid and more economical of operator time. Accuracy of marking remains the same, but candidates are required to make a *positive selection* to indicate 'don't know', whereas under the *Phase three* Lector system this response was indicated by leaving both the true and the false boxes blank. The Lector document-reader simply noted the presence or absence of selections and ignored those item response boxes left blank or with only the lower half shaded in. In the Opscan system (Fig. 3.2) the answer sheets contain a row of boxes for each question. Each box refers to a single item and is numbered accordingly, i.e., 1A, 1B, 1C etc. In each box there are three small vertical rectangles labelled 'T' (true), 'F' (false) and 'D' (don't know). Candidates are asked to indicate whether a particular item is true or false by pencilling in the appropriate rectangle. If they are uncertain they MUST pencil in the rectangle labelled 'D' since the reading machine checks its efficiency by

Figure 3.2 Opscan Sheet (Phase four)

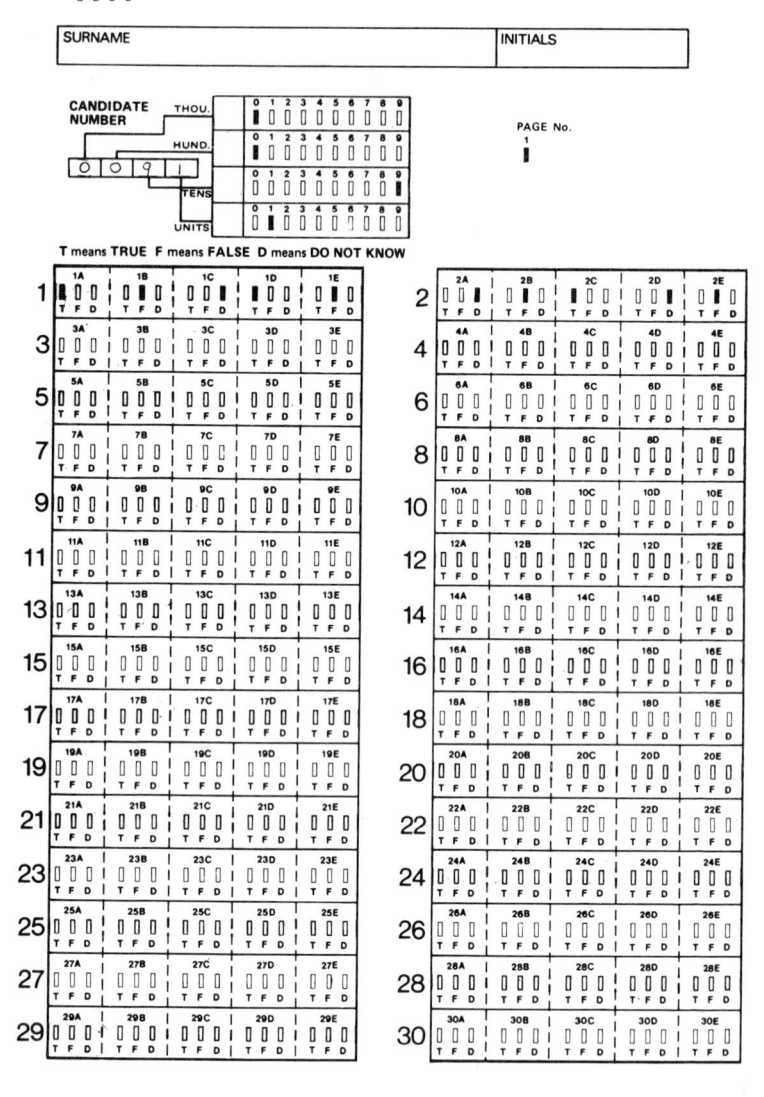

making sure it has sensed a pencilled response for every item. If a candidate is unable to answer any of the items in a question he must fill in the rectangles labelled 'D' for all the items in that question. Thus, he must fill in one of the rectangles in each of the 300 boxes in a sixty-question paper. In the Opscan system the candidate is allowed to change his mind more often than in the Lector system. Selections on the Opscan sheet may be cancelled by deleting the pencil mark with an eraser, and another response may then be selected. This procedure may be carried out more than once since only the most *densely* pencilled rectangle in any box will be read by the reading machine. As in the case of the *Phase three* Lector sheets there is with the Opscan sheets no restriction on the number of true and false items in each question and it is possible for all to be true or all false. However, with Opscan sheets the number of items in a question has been limited to five. This removes the slight weighting factor that is dependent on the total number of items in a question when Lector sheets are used.

All candidates taking MCQ examinations of the multiple true/false type marked by the Newcastle Computing Laboratory now use Opscan sheets to indicate their responses.

One-from-Five Questions

It is of course possible to score one-from-five questions using the various response sheets and automatic marking systems already referred to, although the marking program employed by the computer must be substantially altered. The marking of these questions is referred to in the next chapter. At present, the Newcastle marking program, which is designed for multiple true/false questions, is *not* appropriate for the marking of one-from-five questions.

Alternatively, one-from-five questions can be hand-marked, the candidate simply indicating his selection for a series of questions on a sheet of paper. Scoring is then calculated by the examiner, according to the agreed formula.

CHAPTER FOUR

Marking of Multiple Choice Questions

THE RESULTS OF an MCQ examination should indicate only the candidate's knowledge of the content of the paper and should not be influenced in any way by other factors. This means that a candidate should not gain any advantage by marking questions at random, by marking all his selections true or by marking all false. In these situations he must obtain a score which does not differ significantly from zero; therefore marks are subtracted for items wrongly selected.

Multiple True/False Questions

Hand-marking A meaningful score can be calculated if papers are hand-marked. If the response sheet is of the simple 'right/wrong' type (pencilled response for 'right', no response for 'wrong' or 'don't know': *Phases one* and *two* in previous chapter) the formula for the percentage mark is:

$\left(\dfrac{a}{x} \times \dfrac{100}{1}\right) - \left(\dfrac{b}{y} \times \dfrac{100}{1}\right)$ where a is the *total* number of correct responses made by the candidate and b the *total* number of incorrect selections, and x is the *total* number of 'right' answers in the paper and y is the *total* number of 'wrong' answers. Scores can be calculated by using a grid-type response sheet and preparing two cut-out grid stencils to score the responses, the two stencils indicating a 100% correct (perfect) response and a 100% incorrect response. Each stencil is laid over the response sheet and the number of marks visible indicate a and b when the correct response and incorrect response stencils respectively are used. This marking formula introduces (as did the automatic marking program) weight, depending on the numbers of 'right' and 'wrong' items in the paper. If a true/false/don't know format is used, hand-marking becomes more time-consuming, although any influence of weighting is removed. The marks given for a correct response (whether true or false) are $1/n$, where n is the number of items in a question. Similarly $1/n$ marks are subtracted for each item wrongly selected. Items left blank, or those cancelled without the alternative response being selected score zero. By using this method, scores can be obtained for each question, for every candidate, but in my experience it can take up to fifteen minutes to mark accurately a single sixty-question paper.

Machine marking After the candidates' responses have been read from the response sheets and recorded by the document reader the next stage in the computer analysis is the scoring of the responses by reference to an answer key previously agreed by the examiners.

In the *Phase one and two* formats each question was allowed a maximum of +1, the weighting of the individual items corresponding to the number of items of the same sign within the question. Thus, if p was the number of correct items in a question then $1/p$ was credited for each such item selected. From the sum of these $1/q$ was subtracted for each incorrect item wrongly selected by the candidate, where q was the total number of incorrect items within the question. The theoretical range of marks for any question was therefore -1 to $+1$. A candidate who did not attempt a question (i.e., made no response at all) received zero, as did one who adopted the device of selecting all the items within it. The 'random' score also did not differ significantly from zero since the weighting of positive and negative items was related to the probability of randomly selecting such an item. It has been pointed out in the preceding chapter that this weighting of items is now regarded as unsatisfactory and the procedure has been criticized on several occasions (Harden *et al.*, 1969; Lennox and Lever, 1970; Buckley-Sharp and Harris 1971).

In the *Phase three* format (Lector true/false/don't know) the candidates' responses were read from the answer sheet and transferred to paper tape by the document-reading machine. The 16 photo-electric cells in the Lector machine are sensitive to long wavelength light reflected by the pencilled responses. As the sheet travelled under the reading head the information was transferred in code to paper tape. Because the photocells occupy fixed positions and only recognize pencil strokes lying in given areas of the sheet, the response sheets had to be of standard design and accurately printed, and candidates had to make bold pencil strokes clearly set in the right position. Occasionally sheets were rejected by the machine because they were inadequately, incorrectly or poorly marked. When sheets were rejected, the operator pencilled over as required, corrected errors or cancelled a response which was incomprehensible. The production of the correct tape was the most time-consuming part of the Lector processing procedure and errors in the examination numbers that candidates had recorded on their response sheets accounted for by far the greatest number of problems. The paper-tape output from the document reader was input to the computer.

The *Phase four* process (Opscan) now used is very similar, but here a single photo-electric cell, sensitive to reflected long-wavelength light, scans the stationary sheet, instead of having the moving sheet scanned by a series of fixed photo-cells, as in the case of the Lector. The on-line Opscan transfers its output to a small computer for storage, which facilitates checking, although paper-tape output can be produced. The data on magnetic tape or disk (candidate number plus page number code and pencilled response data) are then fed into the main computer. As with

Figure 4.1 Print-out of Candidate Scores

MARK	%MARK	ST.MARK	%AMENDED MARK
38.00	63.35	1.25	66.79
17.80	29.67	-1.36	31.65
10.20	17.00	-2.35	16.59
24.80	41.33	-0.46	45.13
32.20	53.67	0.50	57.30
29.80	49.67	0.19	52.58
15.60	26.00	-1.65	23.98
27.80	46.33	-0.07	49.83
29.00	48.33	0.09	50.36
36.20	60.33	1.02	63.49

32

Lector, problems encountered at this stage include poorly pencilled responses (mainly responses omitted from the 'don't know' rectangles), although this is considerably less of a problem with Opscan than it was with Lector. Candidate numbers incorrectly filled in on the sheets are still the biggest headache.

After checking that the data now stored on the main computer disk file include that from all candidates, names of candidates together with their identification numbers and any other code numbers to be used for group sorting are fed to the computer from the punched cards. A new disk file is then created comprising candidates' response data plus names married up by the identification number. The answer key is then fed in from cards and compared with each candidate's responses, marks being allocated as appropriate for each question. Finally, the examination results are printed out by the line printer according to programmed instructions. If errors arise during computing, some error message will be relayed to the operator from the computer. Such errors usually involve candidates who have omitted to record their identification numbers on the response sheets, who have recorded them incorrectly or who have used ink or biro instead of pencil.

Calculation of scores The maximum score for a single question using the true/false/don't know format (Lector and Opscan) is +1 and the theoretical minimum −1. Each item is given equal weighting; $1/n$ marks being awarded for every item correctly identified as true or as false, where n is the number of items within the question. For every item incorrectly identified $1/n$ marks are deducted. Using Opscan sheets, where each question contains five items, each item correctly selected scores 0·2 marks and each incorrectly selected is penalized 0·2 marks. Items that were left blank on the Lector sheet or that are marked 'don't know' on the Opscan sheet do not influence the score in any way; no marks are scored if both true and false were marked on Lector or if more than one rectangle is marked on the Opscan sheet. The theoretical maximum for a sixty-question paper is thus 60 marks; this mark is the raw score which is later converted to a percentage and printed out with the raw score. In some examinations the 'standard score' for each candidate is also printed out (Fig. 4.1).

This is computed from the expression $(x - \bar{x})/s$ where x is the raw value, $\bar{x}$ is the mean of all the raw values and s is their standard deviation. This score is particularly useful (and more valid than the raw score) when candidates' performances in a series of examinations are compared.

Weighting of questions It is possible when using the Newcastle Computer Program to weight questions according to their 'importance'. However, preliminary attempts to produce numerical weights for questions have revealed a disappointing lack of unanimity among examiners. The difficulties involved in reaching agreement among specialists on the relative importance of different items of information have been demonstrated clearly by Dudley (1969) and so far weighting has not been introduced in the Newcastle Computer Program. It is, however, possible that weighting of a few questions regarded as being of supreme importance might be incorporated in some MCQ examinations in the future.

Amended Scores

MCQ examinations marked by the Newcastle computer are designed to discriminate between the better and the weaker students and to make it possible to produce a distribution curve for the group which it is hoped will accurately reflect the candidates' abilities. From the beginning, therefore, the discriminating power of each question has been determined in all the examinations marked by the Newcastle program. This is carried out by calculating the correlation coefficient between all the candidates' scores for that question and their total scores for the whole paper. A high coefficient indicates that candidates who did well in the examination as a whole scored well on that question and that candidates who did badly in the examination scored poorly − that question, therefore, discriminates significantly between the two groups. The correlation coefficient is calculated for each question in the paper; all are printed out by the computer. Questions that are too hard or too easy will not discriminate well − those that are too hard lead to guessing or a high 'don't know' response (although the latter will still discriminate to some extent if the best candidates get it right and the others indicate 'don't know'); those that are too easy will result in all, or nearly all, candidates getting the answer right. Questions that are vague, ambiguous or that are misunderstood due to poor wording of the stem or the items will also show little discriminatory power and hence give a low correlation coefficient.

However, even with the greatest care in setting, some poor questions or items may slip through and can easily be identified by scanning the printout. Quite often, the reason why a question has performed badly can be detected in retrospect. Allowance can be made for these poor questions (and, equally, for very good questions with high coefficients) by further calculation and adjustment of the marks. This calculation weights questions so that those with a high coefficient (good discriminators) are given extra weighting and those with a low coefficient (poor discriminators) are weighted down. Thus an *amended score* is obtained for each candidate. To obtain this amended score the computer carries out the following steps:

1. It first multiplies each candidate's score for each question by the correlation coefficient for that question (modified score).
2. The modified scores obtained by that candidate for each question are summed giving the amended score for the paper for that candidate (*a*).
3. The correlation coefficients for each question are summed (*b*).

4. The computer divides *a* by *b* and expresses the answer as a percentage. This is the *percentage amended score* for that candidate.

Examples of how this amendment is done are shown in Figs. 4.2—4.5 using small samples of questions.

It is important to remember that amended scores are only meaningful and reliable when about one hundred candidates or more participate in the examination. The statistical foundations of using the amended mark are unreliable when the number of candidates involved falls much short of one hundred.

The process of using amended scores was originally introduced when examiners were uncertain of their ability to set highly discriminating questions and its purpose was to ensure that poorly constructed questions would be automatically eliminated from the scoring or weighted down (Owen *et al.*, 1967). This was particularly important as there was in the early days (and still is) no means of effectively pre-testing questions before they were used in an examination. Candidates sometimes rightly complained that questions were ambiguous and it was possible to reassure them that if the ambiguity became clear on analysis those questions would have little or no effect on their overall scores. With increasing expertise, the number of poorly discriminatory questions has fallen in most examinations to a very low level. With the highly discriminatory papers now used in most multiple true/false MCQ examinations, the process of amendment has little effect on the result of the examination. The amended scores cover a slightly wider range than the original percentage raw scores but the means of the two distributions are very similar. Furthermore, Fleming *et al.* (1974) have pointed out that in a study on a paper used in the LRCP examination there was no significant difference in the rank order of candidates, whether their scores were amended or not. One possible undesirable effect of using amended scores in postgraduate examinations should be mentioned. Questions outside the mainstream of medicine, such as dermatology, psychiatry and tropical medicine sometimes tend to have rather low correlation coefficients and possibly specialists in these fields, who have answered such questions correctly, have failed to obtain due credit for their knowledge. The time is approaching when the use of amended scores might be abandoned for those examinations that consistently show only a very small number of poorly discriminatory questions.

Short-scale mark conversion It is sometimes convenient to convert the candidates' percentage scores (raw or amended) to a short-scale mark. This may be particularly helpful when an MCQ examination is only one component of an assessment, with other methods of examination contributing towards the total assessment. A method widely used is to define the total range of the short-scale marks and to set the pass mark (previously agreed on the basis of the percentage scores) at 50% of the short scale. One of the undergraduate examinations in Newcastle contributes 40 marks to the overall assessment; the theoretical short-

Figures 4.2–4.5 *Conversion of Raw to Amended Score*
Q = Question number
Score = Candidate's raw score for that question
C.C. = Question correlation coefficient
Amended = modified score (see text)

Figure 4.2 Well-discriminatory paper; good candidate

Q	Score	C.C.	Amended
1	0.6	0.4	0.24
2	0.4	0.2	0.08
3	0.2	0.0	0.00
4	0.8	0.5	0.40
5	0.6	0.4	0.24
6	1.0	0.3	0.30
7	0.4	0.5	0.20
8	-0.4	0.4	0.16
Sum =	4.4	2.70	1.62
Mean =	0.55		

= **55%** (raw)
amended = $\frac{1.62}{2.70}$ = 0.60 = **60%**

Figure 4.3 Well-discriminatory paper; weak candidate

Q	Score	C.C.	Amended
1	0.4	0.4	0.16
2	0.4	0.2	0.08
3	0.4	0.0	0.00
4	0.2	0.5	0.10
5	0.6	0.4	0.24
6	0.2	0.3	0.06
7	0.2	0.5	0.10
8	0.4	0.4	0.16
Sum =	2.8	2.70	0.90
Mean =	0.35		

= **35%** (raw)
amended = $\frac{0.90}{2.70}$ = 0.33 = **33%**

Figure 4.4 Poorly-discriminatory paper; good candidate

Q	Score	C.C.	Amended
1	0.6	0.1	.06
2	0.4	0.2	.08
3	0.2	0.2	.04
4	0.8	0.2	.16
5	0.6	0.1	.06
6	1.0	0.1	.10
7	0.4	0.3	.12
8	0.4	0.2	.08
Sum =	4.4	1.4	0.70
Mean =	0.55		

= **55%** (raw)
amended = $\frac{0.70}{1.40}$ = 0.50 = **50%**

Figure 4.5 Poorly-discriminatory paper; weak candidate

Q	Score	C.C.	Amended
1	0.4	0.1	.04
2	0.4	0.2	.08
3	0.4	0.2	.08
4	0.2	0.2	.04
5	0.6	0.1	.06
6	0.2	0.1	.02
7	0.2	0.3	.06
8	0.4	0.2	.08
Sum =	2.8	1.40	0.46
Mean =	0.35		

= **35% (raw)**
amended = $\frac{0.46}{1.40}$ = 0.329 = **32.9%**

These tables are simply meant to illustrate how the amended score is calculated. The figures are contrived and are not drawn from genuine examinations; only 8 questions are given. For these reasons the differences between raw and amended percentages are exaggerated and no conclusions should be drawn regarding the amendment of these scores other than that
a) with a good paper (most questions discriminating) the range of scores tends to be slightly extended at each end of the range
b) with a poor paper (most questions not discriminating) both the good and the weak student tend to end with a lower amended than raw score

scale range here is 0–40 and the agreed pass mark on this scale is 20. The original pass mark is that decided by the examiners for the percentage range. The formula for converting a percentage score to this short-scale is

Short scale mark =

$$0.4 \times \left[\left(\frac{(\text{original \% mark} - \text{original pass mark}) \times 50}{100 - \text{original pass mark}}\right) + 50\right]$$

The final short-scale mark is always rounded *down* to the nearest whole number; thus 20 remains the true pass mark. Thus, with an original pass mark set on the percentage scale at 45%, an example of mark conversions is as follows:

Original score = 70%   Original pass mark = 45%

$$\text{Short scale mark} = 0.4 \times \left[\left(\frac{(70-45) \times 50}{100-45}\right) + 50\right]$$

$$= 0.4 \times \left(\frac{1250}{55} + 50\right)$$

$$= 0.4 \times 72.73$$

$$= 29.09 \ (\underline{29})$$

Further examples are given below:

Original % score	*Short-scale mark*
80%	32·72 = <u>32</u>
50%	21·82 = <u>21</u>
45%	20·00 = <u>20</u>
44%	19·64 = <u>19</u>
35%	16·36 = <u>16</u>

Provided that the short-scale pass mark is always set at 50% of the full short scale range, this formula can be used for any short-scale range — the only factor that is altered is the first: 0·4 for 0–40, 0·2 for 0–20, 0·5 for 0–50 etc.

One-from-Five Questions

The scoring of one-from-five questions has been discussed by Lennox (1974). As with multiple true/false questions, marks are credited for each correct answer and no marks are given or deducted for an absent response. There are, however, problems with wrong answers, which cannot be disregarded, since otherwise ill-informed candidates would gain marks by random guessing. Most systems in Britain use a 'neutral' counter-mark for wrong responses that is designed to neutralize exactly the effect of guessing. This means subtracting a quarter of a mark for each wrong answer in a one-from-five question; $1/(n - 1)$ marks are subtracted where n is the number of possible answers in the question. Lennox suggests the rather harsher mark of minus one-third for wrong answers but admits that he has no evidence that this is either better or worse than the usual practice. Weighting may be used, particularly when an examination contains more than one type of question, although this type of paper should be avoided if possible. Candidates may accidentally or deliberately select more than one answer to a question. The practice should be discouraged, and it is perhaps best to count any such questions as being answered wrongly, although other much more complicated procedures may be acceptable. Other techniques allow the candidate to indicate varying levels of confidence in his answer, but this also complicates scoring.

Given precise instructions, it is of course possible to devise a computer program that will score the candidates' responses, utilizing either hand-punched tape, or automatic document-readers.

Setting the Pass Mark

The pass mark for an MCQ examination may be based solely on the results of that examination, without reference to any other factors (peer referenced). An alternative (and sounder) method is to lay down suitable criteria for setting the pass mark (criterion referenced). These may be based on previously agreed standards of performance that must be achieved or the pass mark may perhaps be set by referring to the performance of comparable groups of candidates in MCQ examinations of the same character and degree of difficulty. These reference groups may comprise cohorts of candidates who have taken previous and similar examinations, or the criterion group might be composed of an independent body of appropriate individuals who take the same examination and whose scores are used as a basis for setting the pass mark in the exam proper. Both methods are commonly used, but anyone hoping for advice regarding an objective method of setting a pass mark will be disappointed. The truth is that the pass mark is arbitrary and depends largely on the objectives of the examination and the wishes of the examiners. It is sometimes possible and always useful to compare MCQ marks with those obtained in other assessment techniques (e.g., when MCQ, essay papers and orals all comprise a single examination) so that a pass mark somewhat comparable in standard may be determined. This is particularly valuable when an MCQ paper is used for the first time. In future years a similar standard may be achieved by the use of 'marker' questions (see page 44). It is, however, usually advisable to avoid using a fixed figure (e.g. always 50%) for a pass mark in any examination that is repeated regularly with different candidates, such as a final MB examination. This will fail to take into account the differing abilities of various cohorts of candidates and differences in the degree of difficulty of the examinations. The former factor is not likely to be very significant in large examinations, but the latter may be. It is reasonable to devise a pass mark based on the mean of the distribution and its standard deviation (or some fraction thereof) thus providing a cut-off point somewhere on the distribution curve, but this method is only statistically valid if the candidates' scores follow a normal (Gaussian) distribution, and even then the cut-off and the formula used to define it remain arbitrary. Sometimes marks may be presented in grades (e.g. A to F) rather than percentages, but this only increases the problem since as many as six arbitrary decisions now have to be made instead of one, and the procedure does not avoid the decision that must always be made — namely a point on the scale must be defined above which candidates are deemed to have passed and below which they are regarded as having failed. These comments of course also apply to short-scale mark conversion. The only way to avoid setting a pass mark is to take a deliberate decision *not* to set one and to rely not on grades but on percentage or raw scores. The complications that this decision leads to are such that it is a procedure that is not often followed (except possibly in continuing assessment procedures) and the examiner will inevitably find that however long he delays the decision he must usually make it eventually. Despite the statistical sophistication of objective assessment methods, the decision on a pass mark must remain arbitrary and will be the personal decision of the examiners, who will take very many factors into account before defining the critical figure. There is no objective statistical formula that will avoid the need for this arbitrary decision to be made and examiners must simply accept this fact.

CHAPTER FIVE

Evaluation of Multiple Choice Questions

THE COMPUTER MARKING of MCQ yields a mass of data obtained from mathematical analysis of the questions, and these data must be interpreted with caution since it is easy to place too much emphasis on the various indices of discrimination (important though these are) and to disregard the relevance of question content and the degree of ease or difficulty of the questions. Sophisticated statistical techniques, used with judgement, can be of great value in evaluating MCQ. Even so, the wealth of figures thus produced may be too great for easy comprehension and analysis, particularly by those less experienced in MCQ. The relevance of questions must be taken into account by the examining body and particular attention should be paid to the mean scores of the questions that have been set. Relevance of content has already been mentioned (see Chapter 1); the degree of difficulty of a question can be judged from the calculated mean of all candidates' scores for that question. Most computer programs also allow for the calculation of the standard deviation of the mean score; thus the significance of differences between the means scores of different questions or of mean scores for the same question used on different occasions can be assessed. More detailed information about the degree of difficulty of the individual items that comprise the question can be obtained from the figures 'percentage candidates correct' and 'percentage candidates not attempting' (see Definition of Terms). 'Better' questions tend to have a mean score between 0·4 and 0·80 but questions scoring above and below these levels may often discriminate very well. A great deal depends on the objectives of a particular examination, and some examiners will see no objections to including either very easy or very difficult questions if this seems appropriate, always provided that such questions discriminate adequately (otherwise they add little to the examination) and that there is a fair mix of questions with different degrees of difficulty. The balance of emphasis placed on relevance and degree of difficulty on the one hand and discriminatory power on the other must be the decision of individual examining bodies but all these factors should be taken into account in the evaluation of questions.

Discrimination and indices of discrimination have been referred to in Chapter 4, and, unless the examination is simply designed to determine whether objectives have been achieved (when all candidates will be expected to score nearly 100% — see page 14) the discriminatory power of both questions and individual items is of paramount importance. Questions that do not discriminate may be too difficult (perhaps covering a field of knowledge totally unfamiliar to the candidate) or too easy, or may be badly worded, confusing or ambiguous, so that the question or its component items are interpreted in different ways by different candidates. In an examination that is designed to discriminate, the assessment of the questions is as important as the assessment of the candidates' performance.

There are many statistical methods available for evaluating the performance of MCQ (Hubbard, 1971; Buckley-Sharp and Harris, 1972; Lennox, 1974) and many indices of discrimination have been devised. It would be confusing to give details of all the procedures used, which more often than not depend on the marking program adopted. Lennox (1974) gives a particularly useful description of the methods available for the evaluation of questions of the one-from-five variety. The remainder of this chapter concentrates on the indices of discrimination calculated in the Newcastle computer program for multiple true/false questions.

All statistical processes are prone to criticism and we do not claim that the procedures adopted in the Newcastle program are the only possible ways of studying examination results. Refinements to these procedures are continually being made, but in general the techniques used have satisfied the requirements of many active groups of examiners over the last decade. Other examiners, especially those concerned with small class examinations, may be less interested in these statistics.

Evaluation of Individual Questions

The coefficient of correlation between the candidates' scores for that question and their total marks for the full examination is calculated and printed out. A low coefficient indicates that the question failed to discriminate between those who did well in the whole examination and those who did badly; a high coefficient suggests a correspondingly high discriminatory power. It is of course necessary to assess the degree of statistical significance of the correlation coefficient by reference to standard statistical tables. The degree of significance depends on the number of candidates, and the greater this number the lower the correlation coefficient will need to be to reach significance. In some examinations with many hundreds of candidates a coefficient of +0.1 or even less may discriminate at the 0.05 level; with smaller numbers higher coefficients are needed to reach levels of significance. As a general rule, questions with a correlation coefficient above +0.3 may be regarded as good discriminators; sometimes such questions may have been pulled down by a single poor item (see below). Questions with coefficients of +0.4 or more are excellent. Coefficients of more than +0.5 are not infrequently seen, but levels over +0.6 (except in examinations with only small numbers of candidates) are exceptional. In the average undergraduate examination with perhaps 100–150 candidates, questions with a correlation coefficient below +0·2 either discriminate not at all or at only the lowest level of statistical significance. Possible reasons for poor discrimination have already been discussed.

The question correlation coefficient may be used in the process of amending candidates' scores and will be taken into account when the questions are subsequently reviewed. Appropriate alterations will often improve the discriminatory power of a question (see Chapter 6) — even when the question already discriminates well.

Item Analysis

With the *Phase one and two* methods (right/wrong) the method for the analysis of individual items was broadly similar to that used then (and now) for the analysis of questions. A point biserial correlation coefficient was computed between candidates' total scores on the whole paper and whether or not they selected an item correctly. This system was valid since a candidate could only be either right or wrong on each item. However, the system was no longer valid when the true/false/don't know Lector and Opscan sheets were introduced and the marking system altered, since three responses were then possible. Nor was the *phi* coefficient or any of the other established techniques for the analysis of a dichotomy immediately applicable to the new system. An attempt to use the standard (product moment) correlation coefficient was made but was soon abandoned when it was recognized as a statistically invalid procedure; it became apparent that the distribution of candidate scores was usually far from Gaussian, being often clearly bimodal. Another approach that was investigated was to omit the candidates who had scored zero from the analysis of each item and to calculate the point biserial between those who had scored +1 and −1; this proved difficult to interpret as the numerical value required to reach statistical significance varied from item to item depending on the number of candidates attempting the items. Finally, it was decided to calculate the point biserial correlation coefficient using the two groups who were either 'right' (correct) or 'not right' (incorrect plus don't know). This system has proved satisfactory in practice and when compared with the results using the *Phase one and two* marking system has confirmed suspicions of its shortcomings.

With an index of discrimination for each item it is possible to identify those items that are performing particularly 'well' and those that are performing 'badly'. In the process of review of a multiple choice paper particular attention will be paid to the latter (see Chapter 6). The level of statistical significance achieved by the item correlation coefficient can be assessed by reference to standard statistical tables. In practice items with coefficients much less than 0·150 should be considered unsatisfactory (or should at least be subject to critical review), although in large examinations taken by several hundred candidates the cut-off point for acceptability may conveniently be set at 0·100.

In postgraduate examinations held several times each year and with large numbers of candidates the discrimination shown by individual questions and by individual items is remarkably consistent, although occasionally differences may be seen over a long period of time as methods of clinical practice change or knowledge of a particular topic becomes more widespread. In undergraduate examinations with smaller numbers of candidates discrimination may be less consistent; an item or question that discriminates extremely well one year may do so less well on a future occasion, even though roughly the same number of candidates get the answer right. The effect of variations in emphasis in teaching and familiarity may also be observed.

Question Discrimination when Papers are Hand-marked

It is possible to obtain a reasonable idea of the discriminatory power of questions when they are hand-marked, although the procedure is very laborious and is usually only suitable for selected questions where the scores for individual candidates have previously been calculated. The usual method is to take groups of students from the top and the bottom ends of the full scale of marks for the whole examination. The mean scores obtained by the two groups for the questions and their standard deviations are simply compared statistically. Another method is to calculate the *phi* index for the top and bottom halves of the class (Lennox and Wallace, 1970; Lennox 1974):

$$phi = \frac{\left(\begin{array}{c}\text{total score of top half of class} \\ \text{for the question}\end{array} - \begin{array}{c}\text{total score of bottom half} \\ \text{for the question}\end{array}\right)}{\sqrt{\left(\begin{array}{c}\text{total score of whole} \\ \text{class}\end{array} \times \begin{array}{c}\text{difference between total possible} \\ \text{score and actual total score}\end{array}\right)}}$$

A *phi* index over 0·2 represents a useful degree of discrimination.

Clearly these methods are less sophisticated and less accurate than when computer methods are used.

CHAPTER SIX

Revision of Questions and Feedback

THE 'PERFECT' MCQ paper is one where *every* question discriminates at a high level of significance and where each question achieves what is regarded as a satisfactory degree of difficulty. It is virtually impossible to set a paper that reaches these ideals since the great majority of papers contain a high proportion of questions that are being used for the first time and there is no effective way of pre-testing questions that have not been used previously. If a paper were to be composed *entirely* of questions that had been used previously and that met the required criteria without any modification ('markers'), the bank from which such questions were drawn would need to be enormous in order to provide a sufficient number of questions of this type that covered adequately the whole field to be tested in the examination and to provide a completely new paper on each occasion the examination was taken. Even then, there would be no certainty that questions would behave in entirely the same way when they were used on a second occasion (although they usually do). Nevertheless, it is the ambition of every examination secretary to have a bank of used (validated) questions of high quality that would be large enough to allow him to set a perfect paper if he wished. Some used questions will perform sufficiently well to enter the bank unaltered; on the other hand a few will not be worth revision. Many will prove adequate, but may fall short of the ideal — perhaps one item is noticeably weaker than the others; perhaps the question may be just a little too easy or too difficult. These considerations indicate the need for an adequate procedure for the revision of questions after use, since re-use of questions is of course universal. Such revision is necessary so that (hopefully) the discriminatory power of questions might be improved progressively, errors that have passed unobserved might be corrected and, by alteration to the stem and items, an acceptable degree of difficulty might be achieved if a question has been found to be too easy or too difficult.

Marker Questions

Some questions will of course be used more than once in unaltered form. These 'marker' questions are of particular value since by their use the abilities of cohorts of candidates in different examinations and the degree of difficulty of the examinations themselves may be compared. It may be found, for instance, that in one examination the mean score is lower than has usually been found in previous examinations. If the mean score for the marker questions is also lower than on the occasions they were used previously this indicates that the group as a whole was weaker than earlier groups. If the mean score for the markers is much the same as on their first use, the examination overall was more difficult than previous ones. However, marker questions can also reflect changing trends in teaching and increased knowledge of a topic previously not well known. Factors such as these can clearly affect the scores of marker questions and a fair number must be included — at least 8—10 in a sixty-question paper. Consistent and significant changes in the scores of the marker questions under these circumstances can then lead to valid conclusions on the quality of the candidates and the degree of difficulty of the examination. Inconsistent and random fluctuations are unlikely to be significant in the context of the candidates' abilities, or the difficulty of the examination.

Revision of Questions

Assessment of the questions is as important as assessment of the candidates. The methods of evaluating MCQ have been referred to in Chapter 5. The greater the number of people involved in the process of revision the better, since what may seem obvious and clear to a specialist in one field may not be as clear to someone in another field. When questions are reviewed by a committee of examiners there *must* be complete unanimity of opinion. If a single member expresses disagreement or has doubts or reservations the item under discussion must be discarded, or altered until agreement is reached. The answer key originally agreed must be checked and it should be confirmed that the key as printed out by the computer is correct. (The computer will not make a mistake but the proof-reader of the answer key might — in theory; in fact such errors are exceptionally rare since answer keys are so carefully checked. In my personal experience such an error might occur once every four or five examinations — one error per 1200—1500 items). In certain circumstances students themselves can play an invaluable role in the process of revision and validation. In many class examinations in Newcastle the answers are given to the class as soon as the response sheets have been collected, and their comments on the answers and any ambiguity in the wording of the questions are carefully noted. Not infrequently, wording that appears clear to experienced teachers may not be so clear to students, and their comments are often illuminating as well as helpful. Occasionally errors of fact that escaped the examiners will be detected by students — although students can be reassured that such errors will be compensated for in the amendment procedure. Such immediate feedback after an examination can also be a most valuable educational exercise.

Every postgraduate examination and professional undergraduate examination should be carefully reviewed by the examiners when the results are available. Preferably this is done in committee so that all comments may be heard and discussed, although this is not always possible in the case of undergraduate examinations. In this case the paper should be carefully reviewed by one or two individuals, independently or together, and copies of the questions and their analysis should be sent to those teachers who set them, inviting comment. A full explanation of the computer printout should of course also be given, so that meaningful amendments can if necessary be made (those who set questions should also be advised about the form questions should take and reminded of the possible pitfalls discussed in Chapter 2).

During the process of revision, either in committee or by individuals, very difficult questions may be revised to make them easier and very easy questions altered to increase their degree of difficulty. As regards discrimination, examiners are first advised to consider the question correlation coefficient. Rarely this will be so low that no amount of modification will improve matters and the question is then best discarded, although any satisfactory items might be retained for use in another question. Not infrequently the correlation coefficient is so high that any attempt to tamper would be ill-advised — unless there happens to be a single weak item that can be usefully (and safely) revised. In the case of an adequate but not outstanding question, it may be apparent on review that better wording of the stem might reasonably be expected to produce an all-round improvement. The examiner should then turn his attention to the individual items. Sometimes one or more very poorly discriminating items will immediately attract attention and it is these that should be given close scrutiny. Sometimes the reasons for a poor performance will be apparent — ambiguous, misleading or excessively permissive, too great a degree of difficulty or too easy an item. The last two circumstances can be detected by a study of the 'percentage candidates correct' and 'percentage not attempting' figures. Revision or replacement of these items will often improve the questions. Very rarely, a statistically significant *negative* item biserial may be observed. This should alert the examiner to check for a possible incorrect answer key, but more often this means that the best candidates have read something into the question that was not intended (and sometimes may have been overlooked) by the examiner. Such an item must go. It should be pointed out, however, that a low biserial should not automatically disqualify an item if the examiner is convinced that the item tests something that candidates should know. A low correlation may merely mean that for some reason the better students have not learnt anything more about that particular point than the weaker students, although in practice this really applies to undergraduate rather than to postgraduate examinations. Sometimes an item or a question may both score badly and show poor discrimination because it tests an aspect of recent knowledge that has not become familiar to candidates. In an undergraduate examination such a result may point to a particular area where knowledge is lacking and may influence subsequent teaching. In a postgraduate examination it may be decided to leave the question unaltered but to test it again on a future occasion when knowledge may be wider.

Sometimes a question will show a rather low overall correlation coefficient (0·200 to 0·250 or thereabouts) and a string of unimpressive although not catastrophic item biserials. The examiner must then decide whether it is worth while undertaking major reconstruction based on the original or whether it would not be better to discard the question and write a new one. Questions revised in this way are returned to the bank and are usually reviewed again before their use in a future examination. In most cases the revised question will be found to perform better on its next outing.

An example of how an item may be revised has already been given in Chapter 2 (page 18). Further examples follow below:

Example 1 Revision of a question

Original Mitral incompetence is associated with   *Item biserial*

+A. left ventricular enlargement   −0·138

+B. third heart sound   +0·141

−C. paradoxical pulse   +0·213

+D. atrial fibrillation   +0·037

+E. malar flush   −0·075

Question correlation coefficient = 0·081

Revision Characteristic features of mitral stenosis include

−A. left ventricular enlargement   +0·253

−B. third heart sound   +0·257

−C. paradoxical pulse   +0·401

+D. atrial fibrillation   +0·253

+E. malar flush   +0·188

Question correlation coefficient = 0·480

Comment A vast improvement using a more precise stem and the same items (key altered). Note particularly the performance of the three false items.

Example 2 Rewording of stem (some necessitating associated syntactical changes in wording of items; some simply producing a briefer and possibly clearer stem)

(a) *old stem:* 'Glycosuria may be found in patients with'
    revised: 'Glycosuria is a recognized finding in'

(b) *old stem:* 'The following diseases and carriers are associated'
    revised: 'The following infections are correctly linked with important animal carriers'
(c) *old stem:* 'A bullous eruption may occur in'
    revised: 'A bullous eruption is a characteristic feature of'
(d) *old stem:* 'It is sometimes necessary to assist bowel evacuation by various means. The following statements are correct'
    revised: 'In the treatment of constipation'
(e) *old stem:* 'Systemic fat embolism is often associated with'
    revised: 'Recognized consequences of fat embolism include'
(f) *old stem:* 'The following statements about epidemic infective hepatitis (hepatitis A) are correct'
    revised: 'In infective hepatitis (hepatitis A)'
(g) *old stem:* 'The following diseases may lead to secondary amyloidosis'
    revised: 'Amyloidosis is a recognized complication of'
(h) *old stem:* 'A collapsing pulse is likely to be found in patients with'
    revised: 'A collapsing pulse is a characteristic finding in patients with'

Example 3 Rewording of items (all performed better on a second run).
(a) (In acromegaly)
    old item: 'There is invariably enlargement of the pituitary fossa on skull X-ray' ('invariably' is an absolute term)
    revised: 'Enlargement of the frontal sinuses is a characteristic feature'
(b) *old item:* 'vomiting of blood-stained material'
    revised: 'vomiting' (old stem asked two questions)
(c) (Pleural effusion)
    old item: 'is associated with rheumatoid arthritis'
    revised: 'is a recognized complication of rheumatoid arthritis'
(d) (In ankylosing spondylitis)
    old item: 'the hips and shoulders are frequently involved'
    revised: 'involvement of the hips is a recognized feature'
(e) *old item:* 'should never be used in epileptics'
    revised: 'is best avoided in patients with epilepsy'
(f) *old items:* (i) 'anaphylactoid purpura'
                (ii) 'Paget's disease'
                (iii) 'mongolism'
    revised: (i) 'Henoch-Schönlein syndrome'
               (ii) 'osteitis deformans (Paget's disease of bone)'
               (iii) 'Down's syndrome (mongolism)'
(g) *old item:* 'is often found in bronchogenic carcinoma'
    revised: 'is a recognized feature of bronchogenic carcinoma'
(h) (In Addisonian pernicious anaemia)
    old item: 'atrophic glossitis is common'
    revised: 'atrophic glossitis is a characteristic feature'

CHAPTER SEVEN

The Newcastle Computer Printout

THIS CHAPTER IS intended to help those who set and assess MCQ examinations of the multiple true/false type and whose candidates' response sheets are marked by the Newcastle computer. It draws together all of the data referred to in previous chapters.

The computer first prints out the title of the examination followed by the answer key for each question (Fig. 7.1). In this key 1 indicates a true response and 0 a false response.

Figure 7.1 Answer key

```
       ANS KEY
    1  00010
    2  11011
    3  01101
    4  01001
    5  11011
    6  10011
    7  11000
    8  10101
    9  11011
```

The computer then prints out a full statistical analysis for each of the questions in the examination. The question response statistics are set out as shown in Fig. 7.2.

The figures in the top line, reading from left to right, refer to:

1. Question number
2. Mean score — the mean raw score calculated for all candidates for that question. (Maximum +1·000)
3. Standard deviation of the mean score
4. The number of candidates who did not attempt that question
5. The correlation coefficient between the candidates' scores for that question and their performance in the whole examination.

Below these figures is a series of five vertical columns of item response statistics (for items A to E inclusive).

Figure 7.2 Question response statistics

```
16       0.695            0.504           1       0.486
76.563   89.688*  81.063*         75.250*  71.063*  %CDS CORRECT
0.249    0.322    0.175           0.242    0.203    BIS.CORR
9.500    89.688   81.063          75.250   71.063   %CDS TRUE
76.563   5.125    14.500          8.250    9.750    %CDS FALSE
13.813   5.125    4.375           16.375   19.063   %CDS NOT ATT.
0.000    0.000    0.000           0.000    0.000    %CDS BOTH MARKED
```

50

The vertical columns relating to each item refer in descending order to:

1. % CDS correct— the percentage of candidates correct ('true' items are marked with an asterisk).
2. Bis. Corr. — the point biserial correlation coefficient comparing the scores for that item with their performance in the whole examination for those candidates who made the 'right' response and those who were 'not right' (incorrect and don't know).
3. % CDS TRUE — the percentage of candidates marking *true*.
4. % CDS FALSE — the percentage of candidates marking *false*.
5. % CDS NOT ATT — the percentage of candidates marking *do not know*.
6. % CDS BOTH MARKED — the percentage of candidates marking both *true* and *false* (NOT applicable to Opscan sheets).

At the end of the question response data the raw mean score and raw percentage mean score together with their standard deviations are given (Fig. 7.3).

Figure 7.3 Mean (raw) score etc.

```
MEAN SCORE  =   31.16
STANDARD DEVIATION MEAN SCORE =      5.38
MEAN % SCORE =  51.93
STANDARD DEVIATION MEAN %SCORE =     8.96
```

Next follows the numerical list of candidates, which is often also the list arranged in alphabetical order (Fig. 7.4). The scores given are raw mark, percentage mark, standard score (labelled in the figure St. Mark) and percentage amended mark. Sometimes the standard score is omitted. The number of sets of candidate response sheets processed and the number of candidate response sheets processed and the number of candidate cards fed into the computer follow — these may not be the same since some candidates may withdraw immediately before the examination. These are followed by the mean amended score — (the mean of the candidates' amended scores — a — see page 34) and the mean percentage amended score (a divided by the sum of the question correlation coefficients (b), expressed as a percentage — see page 35) and their standard deviations (Fig. 7.5).

The next list is the candidate list ranked in ascending order in whichever way the examiners desire — either by percentage raw score or percentage amended score (Fig. 7.6).

Further lists may follow — short-scale ranked lists and lists printed out in either numerical or ranked order for any sub-groups that the examin-

Figure 7.4 Candidate scores (unranked)

MARK	%MARK	ST.MARK	%AMENDED MARK
38.00	63.33	1.25	66.79
17.80	29.67	-1.36	51.65
10.20	17.00	-2.35	16.59
24.80	41.33	-0.46	45.13
32.20	53.67	0.50	57.30
29.80	49.67	0.19	52.58
15.60	26.00	-1.05	23.98
27.80	46.33	-0.07	49.83
29.00	48.33	0.09	50.36
36.20	60.33	1.02	63.49

ers wish particularly to identify. Mean scores and their standard deviations may be calculated for these sub-groups.

Figure 7.5 Candidate numbers, mean amended score and mean percentage score, etc.

```
NO. CDS PROCESSED =    87
NO. CDS INPUT      =    87
MEAN AMENDED SCORE=   9.043
STANDARD DEVIATION MEAN AMENDED SCORE =  1.924
MEAN %AMENDED SCORE=  49.778
STANDARD DEVIATION MEAN %AMENDED SCORE= 10.591
```

Figure 7.6 Candidate scores ranked by percentage amended score — lower and upper limits of range

MARK	%MARK	%AMENDED MARK
17.03	28.39	25.29
22.47	37.44	32.54
20.67	34.44	32.89
22.77	37.94	33.39
21.40	35.67	33.84
20.83	34.72	33.90
21.93	36.56	33.96
23.73	39.56	36.30
37.80	63.00	65.29
37.83	63.06	65.48
36.40	60.67	65.51
39.57	65.94	68.78
40.40	67.33	70.37
40.50	67.50	71.20
41.10	68.50	72.96
42.70	71.17	73.41
42.20	70.33	74.47
42.67	71.11	75.03
42.97	71.61	77.08

CHAPTER EIGHT

Hints to Candidates

THE ONLY CERTAIN way to score well in an MCQ examination is to know the answers to the questions. However, it is equally important for the candidate to be able to communicate his knowledge accurately through the medium of the response sheet.

Instructions to candidates regarding Opscan sheets Many candidates may not be familiar with the response sheets used in an MCQ examination. Since the technique of completing the response sheet accurately may be rather complex and since it is vital from the point of view of the candidate that he *does* complete it properly, detailed instructions are always given for any examination. Strict adherence to these instructions also makes the operation of processing the sheets in the computer laboratory much easier. Sometimes these instructions are circulated, together with a specimen response sheet correctly and incorrectly marked, well in advance of the examination. This is the case with the Common Part I MRCP (UK) and other postgraduate examinations, and the candidate is asked to bring the instruction sheet with him to the examination. These instructions will invariably be repeated verbally by the invigilator at the time of the examination. In the case of undergraduate examinations the detailed instructions are usually printed on the front of the question paper. It would be quite impossible to give detailed advice on all the available response sheets. One of those most commonly used is the Opscan sheet, marked by the Newcastle Computing Laboratory, and currently favoured by the Universities of Newcastle, Edinburgh, Liverpool, Leeds and Sheffield, the Royal Colleges of Physicians (Common Part I MRCP (UK)), The Conjoint Board, the Royal College of Surgeons of England (Primary FRCS), the Royal College of Psychiatrists and the Royal College of Obstetricians and Gynaecologists. The programme is also used by several faculties of the Royal College of Surgeons and for marking MCQ papers in the DCH examination as well as other undergraduate and postgraduate examining bodies. The instructions to candidates taking examinations in the Faculty of Medicine in Newcastle are printed on the outside of the question paper and are shown below.

    DIRECTIONS TO CANDIDATES
    Each of the following multiple choice questions consists of an
    initial statement (or stem) followed by a number of completions
    (or items) identified by the letters A, B, C, D, E.

You should first put a firm vertical line in the box marked page number on the Opscan sheet using the pencil provided. You should then mark your paper thus:

(1) If you are satisfied that the answer is true you should put a firm, thick vertical line in the appropriate T box (True)
(2) If you are satisfied that the answer is false you should put a firm, thick vertical line in the appropriate F box (False)
(3) If you are unsure and do not wish to commit yourself you should put a firm, thick vertical line in the appropriate D box (Don't know)

N.B. You *must* always indicate 'Don't know' by putting a vertical line in the appropriate box. This means that if you wish to indicate 'Don't know' for a full question you *must* fill in *each* 'D' box for that question.

Note that in every question any number of items may be true or false. To gain full marks *every* item must be *correctly* identified as true or false. An item incorrectly identified will result in a deduction of marks. An item marked 'don't know' will not influence the score in any direction.

USE THE PENCIL PROVIDED TO INDICATE YOUR SELECTION

If you wish to change your mind and make a new selection you should erase your first selection *completely* with the rubber provided. You are then at liberty to select one of the other two alternatives (you *must* select *one* and indicate it — even if it is 'don't know').

The candidate's surname and initials must appear on the answer sheets.

The candidate's surname, initials and all marks must be confined within the appropriate box.

These instructions should be studied in association with Fig. 3.2. In some examinations the candidates will be required to fill in their examination numbers on the Opscan sheet; where necessary, appropriate and detailed instructions are given. In other cases the candidate numbers will be filled in by one of the examiners after the examination.

Hints on answering MCQ of the multiple true/false type

1. *Always* read the question (stem and items) *carefully*. Be quite clear that you know what you are being asked to do.
2. Indicate your responses by marking the paper boldly, correctly and clearly. Take care not to mark the wrong boxes.
3. Think carefully before marking.
4. Regard each item as being independent of every other item — each refers to a specific quantum of knowledge. The item (or the stem and the item together) make up a statement. You are required to indicate whether you regard this statement as 'true' or 'false', and you can of course indicate 'do not know'. Look only at a *single*

statement when answering — disregard all the other statements presented in the question. They have nothing to do with the item you are concentrating on.
5. DO NOT mark at random.
6. DO NOT guess if you simply do not know the answer — you may be lucky but if you are totally ignorant of the answer there is an evens chance that you will be wrong and thus lose marks. Do not hesitate to state 'do not know' if this genuinely expresses your view.
7. Although you should not guess, you should not give in too easily. Take time to think. It is often possible to work out an answer that does not strike you at once by using first principles and reasoning. Think carefully, therefore, but do not spend an inordinate amount of time on a single item that is puzzling you. Leave it and, if you have time, return to it. If you are 'fairly certain' that you know the right answer it is reasonable to mark the answer sheet accordingly. There is a difference between being 'fairly certain' (odds better than 50:50 that you are right) and totally ignorant (where any response would be a guess).
8. It is sometimes suggested that you should go fairly quickly through the whole paper marking down the answers you are certain of on the response sheet rather than slowly and steadily completing each question one by one. This has the advantage that it 'gets marks in the bank' and avoids your being left with several questions to answer (some of which you may know correctly) when time is called. It also allows more time to think about items you find more difficult. The disadvantage of this method is that you may get mixed up and put marks in the wrong place; it also requires a degree of mental gymnastics to consider so many different topics in a relatively short time and to switch rapidly from one to another. Whether a candidate prefers to go through the whole paper indicating the answers he knows are correct and then returning to those requiring more thought or whether he works through question by question depends largely on his personality, his confidence and his familiarity with MCQ. I prefer the former method, but would stress that this is purely a personal point of view and I would not recommend one rather than another. You will know which is best for you.
9. Trust the examiners. Accept each question at its face value and do not look for hidden meanings, catches and ambiguities. Multiple choice questions are not designed to trick or confuse you; they are designed to test your knowledge of medicine. Don't look for problems that aren't there — the obvious meaning of a statement is the correct one. Read the statement. Is it true or false? Either you know or you don't know. If you honestly don't know and can't work it out, indicate 'don't know'.
10. READ THE QUESTION CAREFULLY AND BE SURE YOU UNDERSTAND IT!
11. MARK YOUR RESPONSES CLEARLY AND ACCURATELY!

Bibliography

Buckley-Sharp, M. D. and Harris, F. T. C. (1971)   The scoring of multiple-choice questions. *Brit. J. med. Educ.*, **5**, 279.

Buckley-Sharp, M. D. and Harris, F. T. C. (1972)   Methods of analysis of multiple-choice examinations and questions. *Brit. J. med. Educ.*, **6**, 53.

Castle, W. M. (1976)   Multiple Choice examinations: lessons learnt. *Medical Education*, **10**, 97.

Dudley, H. A. F. (1969)   Objects of objective tests: a theoretical and experimental analysis. *Brit. J. med. Educ.*, **3**, 155.

Dudley, H. A. F. (1973)   Multiple-choice tests: time for a second look? *Lancet*, **ii**, 195.

Fleming, P. R. (1975)   MLQ.: a supplement to MCQ, *Lancet*, **ii**, 601.

Fleming, P. R., Manderson, W. G., Matthews, M. B., Sanderson, P. H. and Stokes, J. F. (1974)   Evolution of an examination: MRCP (UK) *Brit. med. J.*, **ii**, 99.

Gibson, A. L. (1969)   Second thoughts on multiple choice examinations. *Brit. J. med. Educ.*, **3**, 143.

Gowers, Sir Ernest (1973)   *The Complete Plain Words*, 2nd edn (revised by Sir Bruce Fraser) Ch. 5, p. 80. Harmondsworth: Pelican Books in association with HMSO.

Harden, R. McG., Lever, R. and Wilson, G. A. (1969)   Two systems of marking objective examination questions. *Lancet*, **i**, 40.

Harden, R. McG., Brown, R. A., Biran, L. A., Dallas Ross, W. P. and Wakeford, R. E. (1976)   *Medical Education*, **10**, 27.

Hubbard, J. P. and Clemans, W. V. (1961)   *Multiple Choice Examinations in Medicine.* Philadelphia: Lea and Febiger (reprinted 1968).

Hubbard, J. P. (1971)   Measuring medical education. The tests and test procedures of the National Board of Medical Examiners. Philadelphia: Lea and Febiger.

Knox, J. D. E. (1975)   *The Modified Essay Question.* Booklet No. 5. Dundee: Association for the Study of Medical Education.

Lennox, B. (1967)   Marking multiple choice examinations. *Brit. J. med. Educ.*, **1**, 203.

Lennox, B. (1974)   *Hints on the Setting and Evaluation of Multiple Choice Questions of the One-from-five Type.* Booklet No. 3. Dundee: Association for the Study of Medical Education.

Lennox, B. and Lever, R. (1970)   Seminar on the machine marking of medical multiple-choice question papers. *Brit. J. med. Educ.*, **4**, 219.

Lennox, B. and Wallace, A. A. C. (1970) The use of computers in assessment of medical students. *Scot. med. J.*, **15**, 400.

Man Pang Lau. (1972) A theory of multiple-choice examination. *Brit. J. med. Educ.*, **6**, 61.

Owen, S. G., Robson, M. G., Sanderson, P. H., Smart, G. A. and Stokes, J. F. (1967) Experience of multiple-choice-question examination for Part I of the MRCP. Report of a study group of the Royal College of Physicians of London. *Lancet*, **ii**, 1034.

Sanderson, P. H. (1973) The 'don't know' option in MCQ examination. *Brit. J. med. Educ.*, **7**, 25.

Smart, G. A. (1976) The multiple choice examination paper. *Brit. J. Hosp. Med.*, **15**, 131.

Specimen Questions

ONE HUNDRED AND FIFTY specimen multiple true/false questions are presented. They cover the whole field of medicine and include questions on all the major disciplines and most of their sub-specialities. The great majority of questions have been used at least once in medical examinations in Newcastle; all have discriminated, and many have done so at a high level of significance. Quite a number of these questions or their component items have been edited (see Chapter 6) after their appearance in the Newcastle exams. A small number of questions are presented for the first time. The questions are printed on the left-hand page and the answers, together with comments, on the right-hand page. The right-hand page should of course be concealed if the reader wishes to test himself; it has been considered more helpful to place the answers and comments adjacent to the questions rather than at the end since it is hoped that the material will have educational as well as testing value. I hope that few of the ambiguities referred to in Chapter 2 are prominent; if any such occur I can only plead that even with the greatest care it is possible to overlook some of them, particularly when 750 items are presented. Readers can take comfort in the fact that all the questions that have been used before have discriminated significantly at least once, and the great majority of their items have discriminated also. Most of the items that did not discriminate in the undergraduate examinations have been edited or replaced; the only ones retained are those dealing with fundamental and important aspects of knowledge that the candidate really should know. Furthermore, any gross ambiguities (or any answers given that the reader considers to be wrong) would, in a real examination, be compensated for by the process of amending the raw marks.

Readers can obtain a raw score for their efforts by the following steps:

1. Select a series of questions to be answered.
2. Answer them by marking a sheet of paper T, F or D (for true, false and don't know) for each item of each question. (Keep each question separate)
3. Compare the answers given in the book with the answers on the sheet of paper.
4. In each question award 0·2 marks for each item correctly identified as either true or false and subtract 0·2 marks for each item wrongly identified. 'Don't know' does not influence the score.

5. Work out the raw score for each question (the theoretical range is −1·0 − +1·0), sum the scores for the total number of questions attempted (the maximum possible score will of course be the same as the number of questions) and convert the total actual score to a percentage of the total possible score.

Readers will notice that the spacing between the items of the questions is not always regular. This is deliberate, and the questions have been set down in this way so that they line up exactly with the answers and comments, thus making it easier to compare individual items and their answers. Readers can be assured that there is *no* relationship between the amount of space between the items as printed and their answers (true or false)!

Breakdown of Topics

Questions	Main Topics*
1–8	Dermatology
9–12	Microbiology/Infectious Diseases
13–17	Physiology
18	Anatomy
19–26	Pharmacology/Clinical Pharmacology
27–32	Histopathology
33–44	Paediatrics
45–52	Psychological Medicine
53–58	Cardiology
59–64	Respiratory Disease
65–70	Blood
71–74	Gastro-enterology
75–78	Renal
79–85	Endocrinology
86–91	Metabolism, Nutrition and Clinical Biochemistry
92–95	Rheumatology
96–103	Neurology
104–110	Ophthalmology
111–117	Ear, Nose and Throat
118–130	Surgery
131–136	Orthopaedics
137–138	Anaesthesia
139–150	Obstetrics and Gynaecology

* A number of questions cover more than one discipline

1   Erythema nodosum is a recognized complication of

A   sarcoidosis

B   diabetes mellitus
C   Crohn's disease

D   treatment with an oestrogen/progestogen oral contraceptive

E   streptococcal infection

2   The following conditions predispose to cutaneous fungal infection:

A   psoriasis
B   acute leukaemia
C   iron deficiency anaemia
D   idiopathic hypoparathyroidism
E   thyrotoxicosis

3   Arthropathy is a recognized complication of

A   urticaria
B   erythema multiforme

C   lichen planus
D   serum sickness

E   stasis dermatitis

4   Pruritus is a recognized feature of

A   scabies
B   myxoedema
C   Hodgkin's disease
D   chronic renal failure

E   primary biliary cirrhosis

1

A	TRUE	Well-recognized presentation. Look for hilar lymphadenopathy
B	FALSE	No known association
C	TRUE	Should always be remembered. Check on bowel symptoms and examine perianal and anal region in all patients with E.N.
D	TRUE	May cause problems in diagnosis in the female. May also complicate pregnancy
E	TRUE	You should certainly know this

2

A	FALSE	No connection whatsoever
B	TRUE	A well recognized and often distressing complication
C	FALSE	No association
D	TRUE	May also affect nails
E	FALSE	No recognized association

3

A	TRUE	An easy one
B	TRUE	Particularly in Stevens–Johnson syndrome. Also, of course, in erythema nodosum
C	FALSE	This disease is of little systemic significance
D	TRUE	There may simply be joint pain, but swelling, redness and joint effusions are well recognized
E	FALSE	No known relationship

4

A	TRUE	Very easy – but in practice sometimes forgotten
B	FALSE	Not unless the patient has scabies, etc.
C	TRUE	Pathogenesis unknown but may be the major complaint
D	TRUE	May be related to high circulating levels of parathyroid hormone
E	TRUE	Can of course occur in any condition causing chronic obstructive jaundice, including drug-induced cholestatic jaundice

5   Diffuse hair loss may result from

A   secondary syphilis
B   dermatitis herpetiformis
C   treatment with cyclophosphamide
D   treatment with diazoxide

E   a febrile illness

6   Blisters are a characteristic feature of

A   psoriasis
B   acute contact eczema
C   herpes zoster infection
D   pemphigoid
E   barbiturate poisoning

7   In the adult, the following are recognized cutaneous manifestions of internal malignant neoplasia or reticulosis

A   dermatomyositis

B   acquired ichthyosis

C   acanthosis nigricans

D   lichen planus
E   herpes zoster

8   Recognized causes of oral leukoplakia include

A   iron deficiency
B   ulcerative colitis
C   tobacco smoking
D   pemphigus vulgaris
E   syphilis

5

A	TRUE	Very rarely seen now, but a typical feature
B	FALSE	No causal relationship
C	TRUE	Should be well known
D	FALSE	Diazoxide tends to cause *excess* hair growth, which may limit its use in the treatment of hypertension
E	TRUE	Telogen effluvium

6

A	FALSE	One of the few skin diseases which do not produce blisters
B	TRUE	
C	TRUE	
D	TRUE	
E	TRUE	Well recognized. Can be a valuable diagnostic sign in a comatose patient

A very easy question. Any wrong answers should cause concern.

7

A	TRUE	Malignant disease, especially carcinoma, is found in at least 20% of adult patients with dermatomyositis
B	TRUE	Ichthyosis or dry skin may be acquired in wasting diseases such as reticuloses, leukaemia and carcinoma
C	TRUE	Associated with visceral carcinoma. (A similar condition with no such associations — pseudo-acanthosis nigricans — may occur in obesity)
D	FALSE	No association. See comment on 3C
E	TRUE	Reticuloses — a well-recognized complication of Hodgkin's disease

8

A	FALSE	Glossitis and angular stomatitis — not leukoplakia
B	FALSE	No association
C	TRUE	An important association — precancerous
D	FALSE	No association
E	TRUE	Uncommon now but well recognized

9   Faecal excretion plays an important part in the spread of the following pathogens

A   polioviruses
B   *M. tuberculosis*
C   adenoviruses

D   *Shigella flexneri*

E   *Pasteurella pestis*

10   Sabin (oral) poliomyelitis vaccine is preferable to the Salk (injectable) variety because

A   it confers lifelong immunity
B   a single dose of the oral vaccine produces antibodies against all three types of polio virus
C   the virus used in the oral vaccine has been killed before administration
D   Sabin vaccine produces intestinal immunity as well as circulating antibodies

E   the Sabin vaccine can be used for the control of outbreaks of poliomyelitis

11   Tuberculin

A   is a toxin produced by *M. tuberculosis*

B   when injected gives rise to humoral antibodies
C   is used as a prophylactic immunizing agent
D   when injected produces a delayed inflammatory response in a person who is immune to *M. tuberculosis*
E   is relatively heat stable when in concentrated solution

9

A	TRUE	Important to remember this
B	FALSE	Don't be silly
C	TRUE	A high proportion of infected persons have virus in the stool, which may be a source for the spread of infection. Viruria has also been observed
D	TRUE	Of course. Bacillary dysentery. In countries with poor sanitary standards flies are an important transmitting agent
E	FALSE	Plague. Rats and rat fleas

10

A	FALSE	Neither variety does
B	FALSE	Monovalent vaccine protects against only one strain; trivalent produces an adequate antibody response only after two doses
C	FALSE	Live virus strains of low virulence and high antigenicity are used
D	TRUE	Oral vaccine virus multiplies in the intestinal tract and remains at this site. Intestinal immunity is an important advantage — minimal or no multiplication in the bowel occurs on exposure to 'wild' strains of virus
E	TRUE	The widespread use of oral vaccine in the presence of epidemic poliomyelitis may lead to the replacement of the 'wild' paralytogenic strain by the one in the vaccine

11

A	FALSE	Basically a filtrate from a boiled culture of tubercle bacilli. PPD is a purified form but tuberculin is a very constant and satisfactory preparation. (1 tuberculin unit = 1–10,000 dilution $\equiv$ 0·00002 mg PPD; 10 tuberculin units = 1–1000 dilution $\equiv$ 0·0002 mg PPD)
B	FALSE	No
C	FALSE	Used diagnostically (Mantoux, Pirquet, Tine and Heaf tests). Don't confuse with BCG
D	TRUE	Yes. The basis of the above tests
E	TRUE	This is true

12 Characteristic features of typhoid fever include

A an incubation period of about four weeks
B a polymorph leucocytosis in the early stages of the illness
C a macular rash on the trunk
D profuse watery diarrhoea in the first week of the fever
E resolution of fever within three or four days of starting chloramphenicol in appropriate dosage

13 The following statements are correct:

A Altitude sickness may be prevented by breathing oxygen
B In people adapted to altitude the CSF bicarbonate concentration is high
C The 'bends' are caused by bubbles of carbon dioxide forming in the blood stream and causing emboli
D A diver suffering from the 'bends' should be treated by rapid decompression
E Drowning is likely to occur more rapidly during immersion in sea water than in fresh water of the same temperature

14 The oxygen content of the arterial blood is reduced

A by the presence of a left to right shunt in the heart
B in patients with fibrosing alveolitis in whom the arterial Pa, CO_2 is low
C in carbon monoxide poisoning
D in methaemoglobinaemia
E in Fallot's tetralogy

15 The following conditions may result in a raised partial pressure of carbon dioxide in arterial blood

A residence at high altitudes
B gross obesity
C acidaemia due to renal failure
D pure oxygen given to a patient with early respiratory failure
E infusion of sodium bicarbonate intravenously

12

A	FALSE	Variable, but typically 10—14 days
B	FALSE	Leucopenia. Late leucocytosis from peritonitis etc.
C	TRUE	'Rose spots'
D	FALSE	Diarrhoea is late and often inconspicuous
E	TRUE	

13

$pH = 6.1 + \log \frac{HCO_3}{acid}$

A	TRUE	Correct treatment of altitude sickness
B	FALSE	*Reduction* of CSF bicarbonate normalizes CSF pH and allows increased ventilation
C	FALSE	Bends are due to formation of nitrogen bubbles
D	FALSE	Bends require recompression to pressure at which gases redissolve and then *slow* decompression
E	FALSE	Fresh water drowning more rapidly fatal since hypotonic fluid in lungs causes haemolysis

14

A	FALSE	Think!
B	TRUE	In presence of anoxic drive due to defect of gas transfer the Pa, CO_2 will be low
C	TRUE	Carbon monoxide blocks oxyhaemoglobin combining sites
D	TRUE	Methaemoglobin will not combine with oxygen
E	TRUE	Right to left shunt here — reduced arterial saturation and cyanosis

15

A	FALSE	Altitude produces hyperventilation and low Pa, CO_2. Never CO_2 retention
B	TRUE	Hypoventilation (Pickwickian syndrome)
C	FALSE	Elementary
D	TRUE	In this situation the anoxic drive is critical.
E	TRUE	Tests understanding of equilibrium $CO_2 + H_2O \rightleftharpoons H_2CO_3 \rightleftharpoons HCO_3^- + H^+$

16 A low concentration of sodium in the plasma may be causally related to

A   excessive water gain

B   loss of salt
C   hyperlipidaemia

D   hyperglycaemia

E   Addison's disease

17 In a *normal* subject factors determining resting arterial CO_2 tension include

A   cardiac output

B   transfer factor of the lungs

C   alveolar ventilation rate

D   maximum ventilatory ability

E   ventilation/perfusion ratio of the alveoli

18 Complete interruption of the ulnar nerve *at the elbow* will affect the following muscles or movements

A   Flexor pollicis brevis

B   Flexor pollicis longus
C   Flexion at the metacarpophalangeal joint of the ring finger
D   adduction of the fingers
E   abduction of the fingers

16

A	TRUE	Dilutional hyponatraemia (inappropriate ADH secretion, acute oliguric renal failure, etc.)
B	TRUE	Obviously
C	TRUE	'Pseudohyponatraemia'. A spurious reduction in sodium concentration due to displacement of some fraction of plasma water by an abnormal accumulation of lipid
D	TRUE	A solute such as glucose can create an osmotic gradient between cells and interstitial fluid. Water shifts from intra-cellular compartment and plasma sodium falls
E	TRUE	Sodium depletion. Easy

17

A	FALSE	Cardiac output *might* be so low as to restrict ventilation but *not* in a normal subject
B	FALSE	Sufficient lowering of the transfer factor to cause CO_2 retention is incompatible with life and is not seen in a normal subject
C	TRUE	True whether the subject is normal or not, whatever the metabolic rate or the arterial blood pH
D	FALSE	This has little to do with *resting* ventilation, especially in a normal subject
E	TRUE	Always

18

A	FALSE	Supplied by branch from median in addition to a branch from the ulnar
B	FALSE	Supplied by anterior interosseous branch of median
C	TRUE	3rd and 4th lumbricals (acting with interossei)
D	TRUE	Palmar interossei
E	TRUE	Dorsal interossei

19 The following are recognized unwanted effects of the drugs named

A   ventricular fibrillation with lignocaine
B   urticaria with aspirin
C   diplopia with digoxin

D   renal failure with sulphonamides
E   megaloblastic anaemia with phenytoin sodium

20 The following drugs may aggravate or cause gastrointestinal ulceration

A   paracetamol (Panadol)
B   codeine phosphate
C   ibuprofen (Brufen)
D   indomethacin (Indocid)
E   enteric-coated potassium chloride

21 Jaundice due primarily to intrahepatic biliary obstruction (cholestatic jaundice) is a recognized complication of treatment with

A   monoamine oxidase inhibitors
B   17-α substituted testosterones

C   erythromycin estolate (Ilosone)

D   phenothiazines
E   alkylating agents

22 Recognized unwanted effects of propranolol include

A   bronchospasm

B   congestive cardiac failure

C   retinal degeneration
D   tachycardia
E   hyperglycaemia

19

A	FALSE	Lignocaine suppresses myocardial irritability
B	TRUE	A not-infrequent cause
C	FALSE	Xanthopsia (yellow vision) the only recognized ocular unwanted effect of digitalis
D	TRUE	And important. Crystalluria
E	TRUE	Due to impaired utilization of folic acid

20

A	FALSE	A safe analgesic in patients with peptic ulcers
B	FALSE	No effect on mucosa of GI tract
C	TRUE	Particularly when dose exceeds 800 mg daily
D	TRUE	Once more, effect is probably dose related
E	TRUE	Causes intestinal ulceration and rarely stenosis

21

A	FALSE	May cause liver damage, but not cholestasis
B	TRUE	Avoid these preparations in patients with Dubin-Johnson syndrome. Testosterone propionate and fluoxymesterone are the safest androgen preparations in this regard
C	TRUE	Important. Other erythromycin preparations are much less risky
D	TRUE	And widely known
E	FALSE	They have a number of unwanted effects but cholestatic jaundice is not among them

22

A	TRUE	Very important indeed. Do not use in asthmatics. Other more selective *beta*-blockers seem less hazardous in this regard, but are still best avoided
B	TRUE	A definite danger — due to reduction in cardiac output Give concurrent anti-failure treatment in patients at risk
C	FALSE	Not reported
D	FALSE	Causes bradycardia
E	FALSE	Tends to potentiate *hypoglycaemia* in patients taking insulin or sulphonylureas

23 The following statements are correct:

A   Hypoglycaemia is a recognized hazard of treatment with a biguanide given alone.
B   Chlorpropamide is best given three or four times daily.
C   The simultaneous use of insulin and a biguanide is contra-indicated
D   A sulphonylurea may be used to treat early diabetes in childhood and adolescence
E   Lactic acidaemia is a recognized unwanted effect of treatment with phenformin

24 Potassium depletion may occur during prolonged treatment when the following drugs are given alone

A   carbimazole (Neomercazole)
B   probenecid (Benemid)
C   carbenoxolone (Biogastrone)
D   bendrofluazide (Neo-NaClex)
E   phenylbutazone (Butazolidin)

25 Impaired elimination of the following drugs occurs in advanced renal failure and will necessitate dosage reduction when they are used in this situation

A   chlorpropamide (Diabinese)
B   warfarin
C   streptomycin
D   morphine
E   benzyl penicillin

23

A	FALSE	Hypoglycaemia not reported with biguanides given alone (remember the definition of hypoglycaemia)
B	FALSE	Very long biological half-life. Given once daily
C	FALSE	They can be used together — insulin requirements will usually be reduced by administration of a biguanide. Biguanides and sulphonylureas also synergistic
D	FALSE	Never. They must have insulin
E	TRUE	Well-recognized and a major hazard, particularly in patients with heart failure, pneumonia etc.

24

A	FALSE	Not reported
B	FALSE	No connection
C	TRUE	Potassium loss, sodium and fluid retention well recognized
D	TRUE	Should be well known. An effect of all thiazides
E	FALSE	No reason why it should cause potassium depletion

25

A	TRUE	Very important to remember in diabetics with renal impairment
B	FALSE	
C	TRUE	You should certainly know this — otherwise you will make some patients deaf
D	FALSE	
E	TRUE	Often forgotten

26 Characteristic features of acute salicylate poisoning include

A   coma

B   vomiting
C   tinnitus
D   respiratory acidaemia

E   sweating

27 Recognized pathological changes in primary hypothyroidism include

A   fibrosis of the thyroid gland
B   the development of the large Askanazy epithelial cells in the gland

C   infiltration of the gland with lymphocytes and plasma cells

D   a predisposition to carcinomatous change in the thyroid gland
E   the presence of circulating antibodies to thyroid components

28 Characteristic features of Addisonian pernicious anaemia include

A   leucocytosis
B   inheritance as an autosomal dominant trait

C   a raised mean corpuscular haemoglobin concentration

D   an increased liability to gastric neoplasia
E   a recognized association with primary hypothyroidism

29 The following structures possess the capacity for rapid regeneration after damage

A   renal glomeruli
B   hepatic parenchymal cells
C   anterior horn neurones
D   aortic smooth muscle
E   epithelium adjacent to a peptic ulcer

26

A	FALSE	Certainly not a feature. Unless the patient was *in extremis*, coma would suggest that other drugs had been taken in addition
B	TRUE	A fairly constant feature
C	TRUE	Should be well known
D	FALSE	They develop respiratory alkalaemia (hyperventilation). Later, metabolic acidaemia due to toxic effects of salicylates on tissues
E	TRUE	Characteristic

27

A	TRUE	A variable but constant feature
B	TRUE	Typical of auto-immune thyroiditis. Most commonly seen in Hashimoto's disease but also recognized in myxoedema
C	TRUE	Another feature of auto-immune thyroiditis (myxoedema is the atrophic variant)
D	FALSE	No evidence
E	TRUE	Yet another indication of auto-immune thyroiditis

28

A	FALSE	Leucopenia, with multilobed polymorphs
B	FALSE	About 20% of patients give a family history of PA, but no clear mode of inheritance has yet been defined
C	FALSE	The MCHC is normal, but the MCV and MCH are increased (larger cells)
D	TRUE	Presumably related to the chronic atrophic gastritis
E	TRUE	Also with other thyroid diseases and other auto-immune diseases

29

A	FALSE	Unfortunately, but obvious when you think about it
B	TRUE	Fortunately, and equally obvious
C	FALSE	Stop being silly. Think
D	FALSE	No
E	TRUE	Yes

30   The vermiform appendix

A   is poor in lymphoid tissue
B   is rich in argentaffin cells
C   is supplied by an end artery
D   most commonly lies retrocolically
E   is innervated solely by the autonomic nervous system

31   Hodgkin's disease

A   is recognized histologically by the presence of Reed-Sternberg cells
B   may develop into Burkitt's lymphoma

C   may be associated with impaired cellular immunity
D   carries a better prognosis when reticulum cells predominate

E   may be complicated by haemolytic anaemia

32   Carcinoma of the large intestine

A   most commonly originates in the ascending colon
B   may develop from a single polyp
C   may show signet-ring features histologically
D   characteristically metastasizes to the liver before the lymph nodes

E   is a recognized complication of long-standing ulcerative colitis

33   Haematuria in childhood

A   occurs in tuberculous infection only if there is ulceration of the bladder mucosa
B   may be due to ulceration of the urethral meatus
C   when recurrent and unaccompanied by other symptoms should lead to a suspicion of focal glomerulonephritis
D   in nephrotic syndrome suggests an unfavourable prognosis
E   occurring in acute urinary tract infection is usually accompanied by a marked increase in the frequency of micturition

30

A	FALSE
B	TRUE
C	TRUE
D	FALSE
E	TRUE

Quite elementary but important anatomical knowledge

31

A	TRUE	The 'definitive landmark' (Cecil and Loeb)
B	FALSE	Burkitt's tumour is a lymphosarcoma which has been shown to be related to two virus infections (reovirus type 3 and Epstein-Barr virus). Read this up
C	TRUE	Previously positive tuberculin tests may become negative
D	FALSE	Reticular (lymphocyte depletion) variant carries a poorer prognosis than nodular sclerosis and lymphocyte predominant types
E	TRUE	Autoimmune haemolytic anaemia

32

A	FALSE	The rectum is the most commonly affected part
B	TRUE	Papillary or polypoid variety
C	TRUE	A feature of mucus-secreting cell neoplasms
D	FALSE	Lymphatic spread is the most important. About 60–70% of growths have already spread to the regional lymph nodes by the time they come to surgery
E	TRUE	Another easy one. Risk is about thirty times greater than in general population. Risk slight during first five years of the disease but appreciable after more than ten years

33

A	FALSE	Certainly not
B	TRUE	A very common cause
C	TRUE	A thing to remember
D	TRUE	Not seen in minimal-change type
E	TRUE	Simply factual

34 Regarding stridor, the following statements are correct:

A   It is commonest in the first year of life
B   There is a congenital form which typically disappears by the age of two
C   The commonest infective form is due to infection with one of the parainfluenza viruses
D   A life threatening cause is acute inflammation of the epiglottis caused by *H. influenza*
E   A previously neglected cause is milk allergy

35 Respiratory distress syndrome of the newborn is a condition

A   to which premature infants are particularly liable
B   commonly detected in still-births
C   characterized by reduced lung surfactant
D   accompanied by patchy atelectasis of alveolar tissue
E   in which alveolar walls are fibrosed

36 A normal, full-term newborn baby

A   may develop physiological jaundice within 24 hours of birth
B   is more resistant to pyogenic micro-organisms than is a child of school age
C   is more resistant to hypoxia than is a child of school age
D   should routinely be nursed in a room temperature of 30–33° Celsius and a high relative humidity
E   may lose up to twenty per cent of his birth weight during the first three days of life without causing any special concern

34

A	FALSE	Occurs later
B	TRUE	Remember this
C	TRUE	Factual
D	TRUE	Very important indeed. Urgent treatment needed
E	FALSE	Nonsense

35

A	TRUE	This is certainly the case and is well known
B	FALSE	The baby has to breathe before the syndrome appears.
C	TRUE	This is now well known. The lungs of the RDS baby are immature
D	TRUE	A characteristic feature
E	FALSE	Does not occur

36

A	FALSE	No. Jaundice within the first 24 hours would cause anxiety. Physiological jaundice typically appears between the third and fifth days.
B	FALSE	Less resistant. No transfer of passive immunity
C	TRUE	More resistant
D	FALSE	Certainly not necessary in a normal full-term baby
E	FALSE	Certainly not. This degree of loss would cause grave concern. Think what it means in terms of weight.

37 A child, whose birth weight was 4 kg, from the early weeks of life fails to gain weight satisfactorily. She has a very good appetite but is troubled with persistent diarrhoea, with offensive stools. During her second year she developed a cough and had four attacks of bronchitis. She is brought to hospital soon after her second birthday. It is likely that

A she excretes more than 5 g of fat a day in the stools while taking a normal hospital diet
B a jejunal biopsy would show marked villous atrophy
C her sweat contains less than 50 mmol of sodium per litre
D the sputum might well grow staphylococcus pyogenes
E she will improve on a gluten-free diet

38 Characteristic features of nutritional rickets in childhood include

A a raised plasma inorganic phosphorus concentration
B a lowered plasma bicarbonate concentration
C a raised serum alkaline phosphatase activity
D histological evidence of increased osteoblastic activity
E a tendency to spontaneous fractures of the shafts of the long bones

37 If you diagnose cystic fibrosis here the rest is easy

A TRUE   Steatorrhoea
B FALSE This would indicate gluten sensitive enteropathy. The association of offensive diarrhoea, poor weight gain and recurrent respiratory infections suggests cystic fibrosis
C FALSE Sweat sodium concentration increased in cystic fibrosis
D TRUE   A common pathogen in this situation
E FALSE This applies to gluten sensitive enteropathy.

38

A FALSE Low in nutritional rickets, high in certain types of renal rickets
B FALSE Would be low in some forms of renal rickets, e.g. renal tubular acidosis
C TRUE   Characteristic and constant
D TRUE   Osteoblastic activity increases and osteoid is laid down, but the epiphysis becomes broad and disorganized as deposition of calcium and phosphate to produce ossification of the osteoid is poor
E FALSE Bone deformity but not fractures

39 A boy of ten punctures his foot on a rusty nail. Five days later he feels vaguely unwell. Within the next two days the development of painful cramp in the legs and finally of generalized tonic spasms indicates that he is suffering from tetanus

A The clinical picture indicates a severe form of the disease

B Enquiry might well reveal that he had received satisfactory primary immunization in infancy and a booster dose on starting school

C Tracheostomy and positive pressure ventilation will probably be necessary

D If anti-tetanus serum is given, active immunization with tetanus toxoid will be necessary at the end of the illness

E If this boy recovers he is likely to be left with neurological disability

40 The following statements about Lancefield group A haemolytic streptococci are correct

A They are becoming increasingly resistant to benzyl penicillin
B There is a strong connection between infection with this organism and the nephrotic syndrome
C They are one of the principal organisms giving rise to pyogenic meningitis in the UK at the present time
D They may persist in the carrier state in one or more members of a family and give rise to intermittent illnesses over a long period of time
E They are no longer the main cause of scarlet fever

41 Characteristic features of craniopharyngioma include

A papilloedema at an early stage
B over-production of growth hormone by the tumour
C accelerated fusion of the epiphyses
D erosion of the posterior clinoid processes demonstrable radiologically
E diabetes insipidus

39

A	TRUE	Short incubation period and rapid progression to generalized spasms
B	FALSE	Although booster doses are needed every 3 to 5 years to maintain effective immunity, the disease would never proceed as rapidly as this after satisfactory primary immunization and one booster dose
C	TRUE	Related to the severity
D	TRUE	No immunity after an attack of the disease. Active immunization needed and in a previously unprotected patient toxoid should not be given at the same time as anti-tetanus serum
E	FALSE	If recovery occurs it will be complete

40

A	FALSE	They remain sensitive
B	FALSE	No proven causal relationship
C	FALSE	Meningococci, pneumococci and *H. influenzae* are more important
D	TRUE	If one member of a family develops a streptococcal infection the other members should all be examined and treated, otherwise this situation can arise
E	FALSE	Yes they are

41

A	FALSE	Not early
B	FALSE	No hormones secreted
C	FALSE	Certainly not
D	TRUE	A feature of suprasellar tumour. There is also often intracranial calcification shown on X-ray
E	TRUE	Involvement of median eminence and hypothalamus Craniopharyngioma is the commonest primary suprasellar tumour causing diabetes insipidus

42 Nocturnal enuresis with daytime control at the age of five years

A   may indicate an ectopic ureter
B   should be investigated by a voiding cystogram
C   is best treated with amphetamines

D   is an indication for circumcision
E   is likely to indicate severe emotional disturbance

43 Characteristic features of measles include

A   conjunctivitis
B   prodromal illness for 14—21 days before the rash appears

C   petechial spots on the soft palate
D   subsidence of fever when the rash first appears

E   diarrhoea

44 The menarché

A   is usually the first sign of puberty

B   occurs at a median age of eleven years in the UK

C   may occur prematurely in children with untreated hypothyroidism
D   usually occurs at the normal age in children who have had premature thelarché

E   eventually occurs spontaneously in children with Turner's syndrome

42

A	FALSE	No
B	FALSE	Certainly not
C	FALSE	Go to jail. Move directly to jail. Do not pass Go. Do not collect £200.
D	FALSE	Why should it be?
E	FALSE	It *may* do, but in the situation described this is unlikely

43

A	TRUE	A typical feature
B	FALSE	Characteristically the prodrome precedes the rash by four days. Sometimes it lasts a week, very rarely longer
C	FALSE	This occurs in infectious mononucleosis
D	FALSE	The fever increases when the rash appears, and falls when the rash subsides (3—5 days)
E	TRUE	An important feature that is often forgotten. May be related to invasion of Peyer's patches

44

A	FALSE	First manifestation of puberty in the female is usually the appearance of breast buds, together with growth of bony pelvis. Seen at about the age of 10
B	FALSE	In this country median age is 12·9 years. (Range 10—16½ years)
C	TRUE	Hypothyroidism is a rare cause of true precocious puberty
D	TRUE	Premature development of the breasts without other signs of sexual maturation is not uncommon. It is not true sexual precocity and the menarché occurs at the normal age
E	FALSE	Spontaneous menstruation very rare in Turner's syndrome. When it occurs usually indicates mosaic XY/XO, XX/XO or a ring or isochromosome rather than classical XO karyotype

45 Characteristic features of schizophrenia include

A   memory impairment
B   auditory hallucinations in clear consciousness
C   incoherence of thought processes
D   feelings of panic in buses and shops
E   a feeling of being under the influence of an external force

46 Delusions are a recognized feature of

A   delirium tremens
B   obsessional neurosis
C   homosexuality
D   pathological jealousy (Othello syndrome)
E   hypomania

47 Those with a 'compensation' neurosis after head injury

A   show a characteristic EEG abnormality
B   often have a history of mental disorder in first degree relatives
C   often complain of 'blackouts'
D   characteristically improve immediately after compensation is paid
E   may improve following anti-depressive treatment

48 Characteristic features of endogenous depression include

A   feelings of passivity
B   feelings of guilt
C   early morning waking
D   grandiose delusions
E   phobic anxiety (agoraphobia)

45

A	FALSE	Memory unimpaired
B	TRUE	Typical feature
C	TRUE	Another typical feature
D	FALSE	This is phobic anxiety (agoraphobic syndrome)
E	TRUE	And very easy

46

A	TRUE	Well known. Also hallucinations, typically terrifying
B	FALSE	Never
C	FALSE	Don't be silly
D	TRUE	A well-recognized feature
E	TRUE	Delusions of grandeur

47

A	FALSE	No characteristic EEG changes
B	TRUE	Often a family history of mental disorder. Patient may have a past history of such a disorder
C	TRUE	A typical feature. Such symptoms are usually vague and sometimes bizarre
D	FALSE	Some do improve but many do not. Giving compensation is not the simple answer to the problem
E	TRUE	Some of these patients have an associated depressive illness

48

A	FALSE	Not present
B	TRUE	Important. May lead to suicidal attempts
C	TRUE	A very characteristic feature. They always feel worst in the early morning. Risk of suicide high then
D	FALSE	No
E	FALSE	No

49 Recognized causes of general intellectual deterioration (dementia) before the age of sixty years include

A Huntington's chorea
B viral meningitis
C cerebral syphilis
D hyperthyroidism
E bronchial carcinoma

50 The following statements regarding alcoholism are correct

A It is commoner in males than females
B Hallucinations during delirium tremens are characteristically of a visual kind
C After they have been abstinent for one year, patients are able to resume social drinking
D It may be secondary to another psychiatric illness such as depression
E The prognosis is worse in female than in male patients

51 Late onset depressive psychosis

A is significantly associated with senile dementia
B has a good immediate response to anti-depressant drugs
C is not significantly related to physical ill health
D is often diagnosed as a dementing illness

E is likely to have a relapsing course

52 The following are of value in the treatment of manic states

A phenelzine (Nardil)
B haloperidol (Serenace)
C lithium carbonate
D phenobarbitone
E electroconvulsive therapy

49

A	TRUE	Well known
B	FALSE	No reason why it should cause dementia
C	TRUE	Very rare now
D	FALSE	No relationship
E	TRUE	Sometimes overlooked

50

A	TRUE	This is simply a fact, although incidence in females is progressively increasing
B	TRUE	Should be well known
C	FALSE	Certainly not. They must remain total abstainers
D	TRUE	This should be remembered in assessing and treating the patient and in long-term care
E	TRUE	Although less common in females the prognosis is worse

51

A	FALSE	No association
B	TRUE	Yes, but relapse may occur
C	FALSE	It *is* significantly related to physical health.
D	TRUE	Often the diagnosis made is dementia and therefore the patient may be written off and not given appropriate treatment
E	TRUE	Unfortunately this is so

52

A	FALSE	This is an MAOI
B	TRUE	A non-phenothiazine tranquillizer
C	TRUE	Should be widely known
D	FALSE	Doesn't work
E	TRUE	Can be very effective

53 A collapsing pulse is a recognized feature in patients with

A   malignant hypertension
B   osteitis deformans (Paget's disease of bone)
C   patent ductus arteriosus
D   alcoholic cardiomyopathy
E   atrial septal defect

54 Digoxin therapy is contra-indicated in

A   ventricular tachycardia
B   complete atrio-ventricular heart block with congestive cardiac failure
C   atrial fibrillation associated with untreated thyrotoxicosis
D   acute myocardial infarction with multifocal ventricular ectopic beats
E   effort syndrome with tachycardia

55 Pericarditis is a recognized complication of

A   thyrotoxicosis
B   bronchial carcinoma
C   Addisonian pernicious anaemia
D   systemic lupus erythematosus
E   azotaemic renal failure

56 A married newsagent of 44 years has recovered from a first attack of coronary thrombosis, has neither angina nor breathlessness, a normal heart size and a normal blood cholesterol. He should be advised to

A   put water-softener in his drinking water
B   refrain from sexual intercourse for a year after the episode
C   change to a more sedentary occupation
D   remain a permanent non-smoker
E   have an electrocardiogram recorded every three months

53

A	FALSE	Of course not
B	TRUE	Due to the extremely vascular bone acting as a functional arterio-venous fistula
C	TRUE	Peripheral resistance is lowered by a 'leak' in the arterial side of the circulation
D	FALSE	The cardiac output is low in alcoholic cardiomyopathy and there is no peripheral vasodilatation. In beri-beri there is a hyperkinetic circulatory state
E	FALSE	But sometimes with a large VSD

54

A	TRUE	Would probably be fatal
B	FALSE	Not contra-indicated if it is necessary for the heart failure. Cardiac output will improve
C	FALSE	Think. No reason why it should be contra-indicated
D	TRUE	Would be
E	TRUE	No indication whatsoever for its use

55

A	FALSE	Although pericardial effusion may occur in myxoedema
B	TRUE	Invasion of pericardium
C	FALSE	No connection
D	TRUE	Part of multi-system involvement
E	TRUE	A well-recognized complication. Cause not yet clearly defined.

56

A	FALSE	No evidence that this will be beneficial
B	FALSE	Nonsense. How restrictive can you get?
C	FALSE	His occupation is not likely to be heavy and if he can undertake it without trouble he should certainly continue it
D	TRUE	Without any doubt
E	FALSE	A sure way to produce cardiac neurosis and of no possible benefit to the patient

57 The following features are characteristic of pure mitral stenosis with atrial fibrillation

A   a loud first heart sound
B   an apical pre-systolic murmur
C   left ventricular hypertrophy shown by ECG
D   an elevated left atrial pressure on cardiac catheterization
E   pulsus paradoxus

58 The normal ventricular myocardium

A   has the capacity to contract regularly after complete interruption of the conducting system of the heart
B   has an exceptionally high mitochondrial content
C   responds to increased work load by hypertrophy
D   responds to increased work load by hyperplasia
E   is of greater thickness in the right ventricle than in the left ventricle

59 Finger clubbing is a recognized feature of

A   asbestosis
B   chronic bronchitis
C   fibrosing alveolitis
D   fibrocaseous pulmonary tuberculosis
E   empyema

60 Acute viral bronchiolitis and pneumonitis

A   characteristically affect middle-aged individuals
B   are typically secondary to another infection
C   may be associated with the formation of epithelial giant cells in the alveoli
D   often show hyaline membranes in the respiratory passages
E   may be complicated by the development of lung abscess

57

A	TRUE	Absolutely characteristic
B	FALSE	Don't be silly. Not with atrial fibrillation
C	FALSE	Never with pure mitral stenosis
D	TRUE	Again characteristic
E	FALSE	Way out. You're being silly again

58

A	TRUE	Think about it
B	TRUE	This is correct
C	TRUE	Of course it does
D	FALSE	No it doesn't
E	FALSE	It's the other way round

59

A	TRUE	Even in the absence of bronchial carcinoma
B	FALSE	Not in uncomplicated chronic bronchitis
C	TRUE	Characteristic and often gross
D	FALSE	Does not occur here
E	TRUE	Very easy. Can develop very rapidly

60

A	FALSE	Characteristically affects infants
B	FALSE	Is typically a primary infection (RSV)
C	TRUE	This is a histological feature
D	TRUE	Another histological feature
E	FALSE	This does not occur

61 Fibrosing alveolitis is characterized by

A   progressive, unremitting dyspnoea

B   attacks of nocturnal wheezing
C   eosinophilia in the peripheral blood

D   hypoxia with normo- or hypocapnia

E   a restrictive pattern of ventilatory abnormality

62 Bronchial carcinoma is a recognized occupational hazard in the following industries

A   coal-mining

B   manufacture of coal gas

C   the asbestos industry
D   welding

E   manufacture of aniline dyes

63 Characteristic findings in respiratory failure occurring as a late manifestation of chronic bronchitis and emphysema include

A   cyanosis
B   muscular twitching
C   papilloedema

D   systemic hypertension
E   an arterial Pa, CO_2^- of 5·35 kPa (40 mmHg)

64 Recognized causes of a blood-stained pleural effusion include

A   left ventricular failure

B   pulmonary tuberculosis
C   pulmonary embolism
D   rheumatoid disease
E   sarcoidosis

61

A	TRUE	On effort at first, becoming progressively worse until present at rest
B	FALSE	Does not occur. This would suggest asthma
C	FALSE	Not a characteristic of fibrosing alveolitis. Extrinsic asthma
D	TRUE	A characteristic feature. No CO_2 retention. Hypoxic drive may lead to hypocapnia. See Question 14
E	TRUE	Not an airways obstructive pattern

62

A	FALSE	Believe it or not, the prevalence of bronchial carcinoma is strikingly low in this industry. Siliceous dusts do not seem to increase vulnerability
B	TRUE	Also in mining of radioactive ores, refining of nickel, manufacture of chromates and processing of arsenic
C	TRUE	Also, of course, pleural plaques and pleural mesothelioma
D	FALSE	Mesothelioma may be related to this trade, but not bronchial carcinoma
E	FALSE	Bladder cancer is associated with this industry, not bronchial

63

A	TRUE	Would be expected
B	TRUE	A characteristic feature of hypercapnia
C	TRUE	Well recognized. Also increased CSF pressure. Mechanism unknown
D	FALSE	No relationship
E	FALSE	In this situation the Pa,CO_2 would be elevated. The figure given is normal

64

A	FALSE	Blood-stained frothy sputum, but not pleural effusion. A transudate
B	TRUE	Of course
C	TRUE	Yes
D	FALSE	Pleural effusion recognized, but not blood-stained
E	FALSE	Not recognized

65   In a patient with pancytopenia

A   the presence of immature red or white cells in the peripheral blood is good evidence that primary marrow aplasia is the cause
B   examination of a blood film can exclude acute leukaemia
C   generalized lymphadenopathy suggests that the patient has myelosclerosis
D   bone marrow examination may reveal deposits of metastatic carcinoma
E   a history of rheumatoid arthritis under treatment could be relevant

66   Recognized causes of a polymorphonuclear leucocytosis include

A   acute blood loss
B   early typhoid fever
C   acute brucellosis
D   diabetic ketoacidosis
E   pernicious anaemia

67   The following findings would *throw doubt* on a provisional diagnosis of polycythaemia rubra vera

A   finger clubbing
B   itching of the skin
C   a platelet count of 100,000 per cu. mm.
D   an ESR (Westergren) of 30 mm in one hour
E   the presence of a mass in the right loin

68   Hereditary spherocytosis (familial acholuric jaundice)

A   is inherited as a sex-linked recessive characteristic
B   is associated with a deficiency of red cell pyruvate kinase
C   is associated with decreased fragility of red cells
D   may produce symptoms in the first month of life
E   is associated with a red cell abnormality which is corrected by splenectomy

65

A	FALSE	Would suggest marrow infiltration, not primary aplasia
B	FALSE	Acute leukaemia can often be diagnosed on a blood film but can never be excluded
C	FALSE	Hepatosplenomegaly perhaps, not lymphadenopathy
D	TRUE	A possible cause of marrow deficiency
E	TRUE	Several drugs used in rheumatoid arthritis can cause marrow hypoplasia

66

A	TRUE	Should be well known
B	FALSE	In the late stages may get this, due to peritonitis etc. but not early
C	FALSE	No. Neutropenia
D	TRUE	You should be aware of this
E	FALSE	Characteristically a neutropenia with multilobed polymorphs

67

A	TRUE	Would suggest secondary polycythaemia e.g. right to left cardiac shunt, fibrosing alveolitis
B	FALSE	A characteristic feature of PRV
C	TRUE	Platelet count usually raised in PRV
D	TRUE	Usually ESR is not more than 1 or 2 mm in the hour
E	TRUE	Would suggest possibility of a renal neoplasm producing polycythaemia

68

A	FALSE	Mendelian dominant
B	FALSE	A separate entity
C	FALSE	Increased fragility. Decreased fragility in sickle cell anaemia
D	TRUE	May be obvious shortly after birth. Hereditary elliptocytosis is not seen until after the age of three months
E	FALSE	Splenectomy prevents red cell breakdown but does not correct the red cell abnormality

69 a patient is alleged to have classical Addisonian megaloblastic (pernicious) anaemia. The following findings would make you *question* the diagnosis

A   an active duodenal ulcer
B   a furred tongue
C   a history of treatment for major epilepsy

D   loss of weight

E   clear, colourless plasma in the haematocrit tube

70 Recognized features of glandular fever (infectious mononucleosis) include

A   sparing of the tonsillar lymph nodes
B   sensitivity, in the form of a rash, to ampicillin

C   pericarditis
D   generalized pruritus
E   raised serum AST (GOT) activity

71 Portal-systemic encephalopathy in a patient with advanced liver disease may be precipitated by

A   a high protein diet

B   intravenous glucose
C   thiazide diuretics
D   gastro-intestinal haemorrhage

E   oral neomycin

69

A	TRUE	Suggests gastric acid secretion and therefore not PA
B	TRUE	Atrophic glossitis in classical PA
C	TRUE	Suggests anti-convulsant (folate deficient) megaloblastic anaemia
D	FALSE	No reason why you should doubt the diagnosis — this is common
E	TRUE	In PA there is low-grade haemolysis; hence plasma would be slightly icteric

70

A	FALSE	They are not spared — no reason why they should be
B	TRUE	Must be remembered. Don't treat sore throats haphazardly with ampicillin
C	FALSE	Not recognized
D	FALSE	Not recognized
E	TRUE	Hepatitis in most cases as shown by raised serum AST activity. Jaundice less common but clinical picture may still look like infective hepatitis (hepatitis A)

71

A	TRUE	A protein binge can do this and in patients at risk a high protein diet can rapidly produce EEG changes
B	FALSE	Don't be silly.
C	TRUE	Particularly due to potassium depletion
D	TRUE	Due to blood in the gut and a fall in hepatic artery pressure
E	FALSE	Silly again. Used to treat

72 The following factors influence the rate of emptying of the stomach through the pylorus

A acid in the duodenum
B a fatty meal
C the volume of the gastric contents
D the presence of bile in the intestine
E the integrity of the vagus nerves

73 Constipation is a recognized presenting symptom in

A diabetes mellitus
B primary hyperparathyroidism
C myxoedema
D carcinoid syndrome
E chronic pancreatitis

74 Characteristic features of the irritable bowel syndrome include

A exacerbation of symptoms by stress
B an accelerated ESR
C symptoms mimicking those of rectal carcinoma
D rectal ulceration
E a normal barium enema

75 In the nephrotic syndrome

A the prognosis is in general much better in children than in adults
B if renal biopsy shows proliferative glomerulitis, a good response to steroids can be expected
C it is hazardous to use frusemide (Lasix) to reduce oedema
D troxidone (Tridione) administration is a possible aetiological factor
E a raised blood cholesterol concentration is a characteristic finding

72

A	TRUE	Causes inhibition of gastric emptying
B	TRUE	Fats delay gastric emptying whereas proteins and carbohydrates are rapidly evacuated if in a suitable physical state
C	TRUE	The larger the initial volume of gastric contents the more rapid the initial rate of emptying
D	FALSE	No effect
E	TRUE	No comment necessary

73

A	FALSE	Possibly nocturnal diarrhoea (autonomic neuropathy) but not constipation
B	TRUE	A well recognized feature
C	TRUE	Well recognized
D	FALSE	Causes diarrhoea
E	FALSE	If symptoms are produced, more likely to be diarrhoea (steatorrhoea)

74

A	TRUE	Characteristic
B	FALSE	Would suggest ulcerative colitis, Crohn's or carcinoma
C	TRUE	This must be excluded
D	FALSE	See comment on **B**
E	TRUE	A *sine qua non*

75

A	TRUE	Simply a fact
B	FALSE	Minimal change lesions indicate prospect of good response to steroids
C	FALSE	Why should it be? Fairly standard therapy
D	TRUE	Should be remembered. May also be caused by mercurials
E	TRUE	Characteristic

76 Urine microscopy would be expected to reveal numerous red cell casts in

A pyelonephritis
B acute post streptococcal glomerulonephritis
C minimal change glomerulonephritis
D analgesic nephropathy
E membranous glomerulonephritis

77 A man of forty has polycystic kidneys, a blood pressure of 180/120, a blood urea of 43 mmol/l (258 mg/100 ml) and a creatinine clearance of 7·2 l/24 h (5 ml/minute)

A He is more likely to suffer a subarachnoid haemorrhage than a patient with essential hypertension of the same severity
B His sons may suffer from polycystic disease but his daughters will escape
C Without dialysis or transplantation he is unlikely to live more than a few weeks
D He should be given a low protein, high calorie, low salt diet
E If he has osteomalacia of the spine with hypocalcaemia he should be treated with vitamin D

78 A woman of twenty-four who is fourteen weeks pregnant and who has no history of previous illness and no urinary symptoms attends an antenatal clinic. Routine MSU culture yields 100,000+ *E. coli* per ml and repeat culture gives the same result

A If left untreated she has about a 25% chance of developing acute pyelonephritis during pregnancy
B The organism is unlikely to be sensitive to sulphonamides
C Treatment with tetracyclines should be avoided as they affect the bones and teeth of the fetus
D If the infection is eliminated by a one-week course of antibacterial therapy and does not recur during pregnancy, it is unlikely that she has chronic pyelonephritis
E Intravenous pyelogram should be performed as soon as possible after delivery

76

A	FALSE	Pus cells and possibly a few red cells. Not red cell casts
B	TRUE	Characteristic
C	FALSE	Not found
D	FALSE	Sterile pyuria
E	FALSE	Not found

77

A	TRUE	About one fifth of such patients have intracranial aneurysms
B	FALSE	The adult variety is inherited as a Mendelian dominant trait, not sex-linked
C	FALSE	The disease progresses relatively slowly
D	TRUE	Appropriate therapy for a patient with azotaemic renal failure
E	TRUE	Osteomalacia is a recognized complication of chronic renal failure and would normally be treated by vitamin D

78

A	TRUE	This is the approximate risk of acute pyelonephritis developing in a patient with asymptomatic bacteruria
B	FALSE	The likelihood is that it would be sensitive
C	TRUE	Tetracyclines discolour teeth and may impair bone growth
D	TRUE	If it clears with no relapse it is unlikely that she has chronic pyelonephritis or any other structural abnormality of the urinary tract
E	FALSE	The dilatation of ureters and renal pelves that occurs during pregnancy takes several weeks to disappear and in the early days of the puerperium will certainly cause difficulty in interpretation

79 Recognized features of anorexia nervosa include

A selective exclusion of protein from the diet

B raised serum gonadotrophin concentrations

C equal incidence in males and females

D hypokalaemia

E lethargy

80 In a previously stable insulin-dependent diabetic the daily dose of insulin is likely to need increasing if

A chronic renal failure develops

B treatment with propranolol is required

C the patient develops thyrotoxicosis

D successful pituitary ablation is performed for retinopathy

E the patient is in the third trimester of pregnancy

81 Oral contraceptives containing oestrogen and progestogen

A cause a rise in the serum protein bound iodine concentration

B may cause increased facial pigmentation

C prevent ovulation by a direct effect on the ovaries

D are much more likely to cause venous thromboembolism in the second year of their use than in the first year

E may impair glucose tolerance

79

A	FALSE	Such patients selectively exclude carbohydrate rather than protein and the clinical picture is very different from protein deficiency
B	FALSE	The characteristic endocrine feature is isolated gonadotrophin deficiency due to hypothalamic dysfunction
C	FALSE	The reported ratio of males to females is 1:10—15
D	TRUE	May be due to secondary aldosteronism but more commonly due to laxative abuse. Contributes to muscular weakness
E	FALSE	These patients are typically hyperactive

80

A	FALSE	There is increased insulin sensitivity in the presence of renal failure
B	FALSE	No increase in insulin resistance. *Beta*-blockers tend to potentiate hypoglycaemia
C	TRUE	Increasing resistance to insulin with weight loss and suspicion of loss of control may conceal the true cause in this situation
D	FALSE	Increased insulin sensitivity is usual after pituitary ablation
E	TRUE	The usual course is for insulin requirements to increase substantially in the third trimester

81

A	TRUE	Due to increased serum thyroxine binding globulin concentrations
B	TRUE	Chloasma. As sometimes seen in pregnancy
C	FALSE	Effect is to suppress pituitary gonadotrophins
D	FALSE	Risk the same throughout
E	TRUE	May precipitate diabetes in a potential or latent diabetic

82 In acromegaly

A there is characteristically enlargement of the frontal sinuses
B increased insulin resistance is usual
C painful paraesthesiae in median nerve distribution are a recognized associated feature
D homonymous hemianopia is the most characteristic visual complication
E galactorrhoea may be a presenting symptom in the female

83 Hypoglycaemia

A may produce visual symptoms without loss of consciousness
B occurs when a normal person fasts for 48 hours
C is a recognized feature of untreated thyrotoxicosis
D is a characteristic feature of hypothermia
E may be responsible for coma in a patient with adrenal insufficiency

84 Characteristic features of Cushing's syndrome include

A generalized obesity
B hypotension
C menorrhagia
D proximal muscle weakness
E osteomalacia

85 The following statements are correct

A In hyperthyroidism due to Graves' disease the serum TSH concentration is characteristically elevated
B Hyperthyroidism in children is best treated by early subtotal thyroidectomy
C Overtreatment of hyperthyroidism with antithyroid drugs may result in an increase in goitre size
D The symptoms and signs of hyperthyroidism may to some extent be alleviated by administration of propranolol
E A scan of the thyroid after oral radioactive iodine will differentiate between a benign and a malignant nodule

82

A	TRUE	Part of the generalized skeletal overgrowth
B	TRUE	Characteristic of active acromegaly
C	TRUE	Carpal tunnel syndrome is a frequent complication (also complicates untreated myxoedema)
D	FALSE	Bitemporal hemianopia is the characteristic field defect in patients with pituitary tumours
E	TRUE	May also occur in males

83

A	TRUE	Diplopia, blurring of vision etc.
B	FALSE	It does not. Fasting hypoglycaemia is characteristic of islet cell tumour
C	FALSE	No. High peak blood glucose likely to be found during GTT due to rapid absorption of glucose
D	FALSE	If anything, hyperglycaemia is more likely due to pancreatitis
E	TRUE	Very important. May be life-saving to remember this

84

A	FALSE	Truncal obesity. Limbs thin
B	FALSE	Hypertension
C	FALSE	Amenorrhoea likely
D	TRUE	A consistent finding
E	FALSE	Osteoporosis characteristic

85

A	FALSE	TSH normal or low, fails to rise after injection of TRH
B	FALSE	Best avoided in adolescence. Treat with antithyroid drugs and delay operation until after puberty
C	TRUE	Suppressed thyroid hormone levels leading to increased TSH drive
D	TRUE	*Beta*-blockers will alleviate many signs and symptoms but best used in association with antithyroid drugs
E	FALSE	A scan will not differentiate reliably

86 Characteristic features of severe scurvy include

A follicular hyperkeratosis
B peripheral neuropathy
C 'magenta tongue'
D macrocytic anaemia
E increased capillary fragility

87 The serum alkaline phosphatase activity is characteristically raised in

A senile osteoporosis
B intrahepatic cholestasis

C extensive Paget's disease of bone
D osteomalacia due to anticonvulsants
E multiple myeloma

88 In obesity

A hypertriglyceridaemia is rare in the absence of diabetes
B right ventricular failure is a recognized complication

C the mobilization of fatty acids from adipose tissue is characteristically impaired
D life expectation is reduced in direct relationship to the degree of obesity
E a raised fasting serum insulin concentration is a recognized feature

89 The serum protein bound iodine concentration is affected by

A paracetamol administration

B administration of an oestrogen-containing oral contraceptive
C ingestion of clioquinol (Entero-Vioform)
D spironolactone (Aldactone) administration
E a myelogram five years previously

86

A	TRUE	Characteristic
B	FALSE	Not in pure vitamin C deficiency
C	FALSE	Riboflavin deficiency
D	TRUE	Macrocytosis common. Returns to normal after treatment
E	TRUE	Well known

87

A	FALSE	Normal
B	TRUE	Characteristic of intrahepatic or extrahepatic biliary obstruction
C	TRUE	Absolutely characteristic
D	TRUE	As in other forms of osteomalacia
E	FALSE	Not a characteristic feature – usually normal

88

A	FALSE	Characteristic of obesity whether diabetes is present or not
B	TRUE	Alveolar underventilation (Pickwickian syndrome) leading to cor pulmonale
C	FALSE	Not impaired
D	TRUE	The fatter the person, the shorter the life expectancy. See insurance statistics
E	TRUE	Insulin resistance with hypersecretion common in obesity

89

A	FALSE	No effect. But salicylates compete for binding sites on thyroid-hormone binding protein and may lead to a low PBI
B	TRUE	Increased thyroid-hormone binding protein – PBI rises
C	TRUE	This compound contains iodine – PBI rises
D	FALSE	No effect
E	TRUE	Raised PBI – effect lasts for years, possibly indefinitely. Media used for bronchography may have the same effect whereas media used for IVP have a much shorter effect on the PBI (rapidly excreted by kidneys)

90 Secondary amyloidosis is a recognized complication of

A paraplegia
B leprosy
C osteoarthrosis
D rheumatoid arthritis
E multiple myeloma

91 Serum creatine phosphotransferase (creatine phosphokinase; CPK) activity is characteristically elevated

A twenty-four hours after a myocardial infarction

B in osteomalacia
C in untreated thyrotoxicosis

D in polymyalgia rheumatica

E in haemolysed blood

92 Ankylosing spondylitis

A occurs most commonly in women over the age of forty
B is significantly associated with the presence of the HLA-B27 antigen
C may present as sciatica
D may be complicated by arthropathy affecting the hips
E may be complicated by iritis

93 Heberden's nodes

A may be caused by trauma
B are a recognized finding in infective endocarditis
C are more common in overweight patients than in the lean
D occur typically over the base of the terminal phalanges
E are significantly associated with a positive Rose-Waaler test

90

A	TRUE	A common complication – often forgotten
B	TRUE	One of the commonest causes of death is renal failure due to amyloidosis
C	FALSE	Does not occur
D	TRUE	In longstanding R.A.
E	TRUE	Well recognized

91

A	TRUE	Rises early, reaching peak at about 24 hours after M.I. Normal by 72 hours (AST peaks at 48 hours and returns to normal by 5 days, LDH rise occurs later and is elevated longer)
B	FALSE	No. Alkaline phosphatase, yes
C	FALSE	A rise may sometimes occur in hypothyroidism but is not very helpful diagnostically
D	FALSE	No. An important feature which distinguishes between polymyalgia rheumatica and polymyositis
E	FALSE	No rise following haemolysis – CPK is not present in erythrocytes

92

A	FALSE	About 90% of cases in men, onset typically in late teens and early twenties
B	TRUE	An invaluable diagnostic test
C	TRUE	Well recognized
D	TRUE	Arthritis of peripheral joints well recognized
E	TRUE	About 10–15% of patients

93

A	TRUE	They may
B	FALSE	Osler's nodes here
C	FALSE	They are not
D	TRUE	This is the characteristic site
E	FALSE	No association with rheumatoid

94 The following are recognized associations of Sjögren's syndrome

A rheumatoid arthritis
B renal tubular acidosis

C xerostoma
D exophthalmos
E salivary gland swelling

95 The following statements are correct

A Hip joint disease may present as pain in the knee

B A normal joint contains so little synovial fluid that the clinical demonstration of fluid in a joint always implies an abnormality
C Joint disease alone is seldom a cause of gross muscle wasting

D A positive 'patellar-tap' test is a sign of patello-femoral arthritis
E Carpal tunnel syndrome typically remits during pregnancy

96 Paralysis of cervical sympathetic innervation results in

A dilatation of the pupil on the affected side
B loss of taste sensation over the anterior two-thirds of the tongue

C partial ptosis on the same side
D dryness of the mouth

E absence of thermal sweating on the same side of the face

94

A	TRUE	R.A. a well-recognized association
B	TRUE	An important association. May be due to deposition of immune complexes around renal tubules
C	TRUE	A dry mouth is characteristic
D	FALSE	Not recognized
E	TRUE	A common feature

95

A	TRUE	A common trap. Pain in the knee may be so prominent that the disease in the affected hip is overlooked
B	TRUE	An effusion is always significant
C	FALSE	There may be extensive wasting in relation to an arthritic joint
D	FALSE	It is a sign of fluid in the knee joint
E	FALSE	It typically gets worse (and may present) during pregnancy

96

A	FALSE	The pupil is constricted — sympathetic stimulation dilates
B	FALSE	Taste over anterior two-thirds of tongue mediated by lingual nerve → chorda tympani → geniculate ganglion. Posterior one-third via glossopharyngeal nerve
C	TRUE	Remember Horner's syndrome
D	FALSE	The parasympathetic fibres are secretomotor and autonomic nerve supply to salivary glands is via glossopharyngeal (parotid) and chorda tympani (submaxillary and sublingual)
E	TRUE	Cervical sympathectomy may be carried out in severe hyperhidrosis

97 The following statements are correct

A Lumbar puncture should be performed in all suspected cases of brain tumour
B The CSF is characteristically normal in patients with trigeminal neuralgia
C An elevation of the CSF protein above a level of 1·5 g per litre is to be expected in motor neurone disease
D An elevation of the CSF protein is a recognized feature of untreated myxoedema
E The CSF cell count may be increased in multiple sclerosis

98 Neck stiffness with occipital pain on attempted neck flexion may result from

A pneumonia in childhood
B post-infective polyneuropathy
C subarachnoid haemorrhage
D posterior fossa tumour
E cervical invertebral disk prolapse

99 Recognized features of motor neurone disease include

A nystagmus
B dysphagia
C muscle fasciculation
D retention of urine
E extensor plantar responses

100 On examination of the visual fields

A bitemporal hemianopia is indicative of chiasmatic compression
B the finding of a right homonymous hemianopia would be consistent with a space-occupying lesion in the left occipital lobe
C bilateral concentric constriction of the fields can only be due to hysteria
D a central scotoma is consistent with a lesion of the lateral geniculate body
E an upper quadrantic homonymous defect would suggest a temporal lobe lesion

97

A	FALSE	Try explaining to the coroner
B	TRUE	It is
C	FALSE	Not to be expected
D	TRUE	A feature of interest but unhelpful diagnostically
E	TRUE	There may be a mononuclear pleocytosis of up to 200–300 cells in the acute disease

98

A	TRUE	Meningism
B	FALSE	No reason why it should
C	TRUE	No excuses for getting this wrong
D	TRUE	A typical feature
E	TRUE	To be remembered

99

A	FALSE	Does not occur
B	TRUE	Bulbar palsy
C	TRUE	A typical feature
D	FALSE	Does not occur
E	TRUE	Typically (although not exclusively) with absent knee jerks

100

A	TRUE	The characteristic field defect in pituitary tumour
B	TRUE	It would be (remember the visual pathways)
C	FALSE	This could be due to papilloedema (usually with enlargement of the blind spot) or glaucoma. Hysteria typically produces apparent blindness, or tubular vision
D	FALSE	Due to an inflammatory or compressive lesion of the optic nerve
E	TRUE	See comment on B

101 In the syndrome of carpal tunnel compression

A   the symptoms are more severe during the night
B   men are more commonly affected than women
C   wasting of the hypothenar eminence is a recognized feature
D   the syndrome may be an early feature of rheumatoid arthritis
E   Addison's disease is a recognized association

102 Parkinson's disease is characterized by

A   increased pigmentation of the substantia nigra

B   a festinant gait
C   cogwheel rigidity
D   bradykinesis
E   an intention tremor

103 Characteristic features of petit mal include

A   a focal structural lesion of the cerebral cortex
B   a normal EEG

C   onset before puberty
D   aminoaciduria
E   episodes of psychopathic behaviour

104 In a child with a right convergent concomitant squint the following statements are correct

A   The left eye will be amblyopic

B   If he is of pre-school age he is likely to grow out of it leaving no sequelae

C   He will have a squint the degree of which remains constant in all directions of gaze

D   A hypermetropic refractive error will be expected

E   The squinting eye may harbour a retinoblastoma

101

A	TRUE	A typical and distressing feature. Helped by night splints
B	FALSE	Women affected more often
C	FALSE	Ulnar nerve supplies hypothenar eminence
D	TRUE	It may be
E	FALSE	Hypothyroidism, acromegaly yes — Addison's disease no

102

A	FALSE	There is degeneration of the substantia nigra neurones, but not increased pigmentation
B	TRUE	Absolutely characteristic
C	TRUE	See B
D	TRUE	See B
E	FALSE	This does not occur

103

A	FALSE	Very rare
B	FALSE	Typically wave-and-spike pattern or a three-per-second wave. May only be present after over-ventilation
C	TRUE	A fact
D	FALSE	Nonsense
E	FALSE	Not in petit mal

104

A	FALSE	Suppression of vision (amblyopia) occurs only in the squinting eye
B	FALSE	No child of whatever age should be left to 'grow out of' a squint
C	TRUE	
D	TRUE	Most convergent squints are associated with a hypermetropic error
E	TRUE	Squints may originally develop due to poor vision in the eye with the tumour

105 Diplopia is a recognized feature of

A retrobulbar neuritis
B Horner's syndrome
C myasthenia gravis
D cerebellar hemisphere lesions
E brain stem lesions

106 Acute (narrow angle) glaucoma is characterized by

A ocular pain
B conjunctival injection
C oedema of the eyelids
D halo vision
E a miotic pupil

107 There is a recognized association between anterior uveitis and

A sickle cell disease
B rheumatoid arthritis
C ankylosing spondylitis
D sarcoidosis
E gonorrhoea

108 Recognized ocular changes in diabetes mellitus include

A new vessel formation in the iris
B looping of retinal veins
C macular oedema
D subluxation of the lens
E secondary glaucoma

109 Recognized features of thyroid eye disease include

A corneal oedema
B infiltration of extra-ocular muscles with lymphocytes
C ptosis
D conjunctival irritation
E orbital fat herniation into the eyelids

105

A	FALSE	No
B	FALSE	Never
C	TRUE	Variable in severity; characteristically begins in the evening and gets worse then
D	FALSE	Why should they? Nystagmus, skew deviation and weakness of conjugate deviation only
E	TRUE	This is where the action is

106

A	TRUE	A constant feature
B	TRUE	Don't dismiss it as conjunctivitis
C	FALSE	Does not occur
D	TRUE	Also rainbow vision
E	FALSE	Typically semi-dilated and fixed

107

A	FALSE	Not reported
B	TRUE	Well recognized
C	TRUE	Yes
D	TRUE	May be severe (uveo-parotid fever)
E	TRUE	Also with Reiter's syndrome

108

A	TRUE	Rubeosis iridis
B	TRUE	An early feature
C	TRUE	An important cause of visual impairment
D	FALSE	Not unless the patient also has Marfan's syndrome
E	TRUE	Secondary to A

109

A	FALSE	Does not occur
B	TRUE	Characteristic
C	FALSE	Lid retraction occurs
D	TRUE	Grittiness and soreness a common complaint, may be chemosis
E	TRUE	This occurs

110 Visual loss of sudden onset can be caused by

A   cranial arteritis
B   central retinal vein thrombosis
C   tobacco amblyopia
D   retinal detachment
E   open angle glaucoma

111 A patient complains of intermittent earache for four weeks, without hearing loss. These symptoms are consistent with

A   an impacted wisdom tooth
B   acute otitis media
C   peritonsillitis
D   carcinoma of the hypopharynx
E   acute sinusitis

112 Otosclerosis is

A   a recognized association of osteogenesis imperfecta (fragilitas ossium)
B   a disease confined to patients over the age of sixty
C   a recognized cause of conductive deafness
D   helped by stapedectomy and prosthetic replacement
E   non-hereditary

113 Recognized indications for adenoidectomy include

A   recurring tonsillitis
B   recurring deafness
C   stammering
D   asthma
E   mouth breathing

114 In carcinoma of the vocal cord

A   hoarseness is the characteristic presenting symptom
B   the disease is more commonly found in females
C   lymph node involvement occurs early
D   haemoptysis is a characteristic feature
E   local pain is a constant feature

110

A	TRUE	The most important complication of cranial arteritis
B	TRUE	Diagnosed on fundoscopy
C	FALSE	Visual loss, but not sudden
D	TRUE	Obviously
E	FALSE	Slow onset

111

A	TRUE	Of course
B	FALSE	Not acute otitis media, or chronic either
C	TRUE	Always examine the throat
D	TRUE	Important to remember this
E	FALSE	Not a feature

112

A	TRUE	Well recognized. Tympanic membrane may be blue
B	FALSE	Usually begins in early adult life
C	TRUE	Easy
D	TRUE	Good to excellent results in over 90% of patients
E	FALSE	Usually inherited as a dominant with up to 40% penetrance

113

A	FALSE	Tonsillectomy here
B	TRUE	A clear indication
C	FALSE	Certainly not
D	FALSE	Never
E	TRUE	Another clear indication

114

A	TRUE	It is — remember this
B	FALSE	More common in males
C	FALSE	A late feature
D	FALSE	Not characteristic
E	FALSE	It is not, until the terminal stages

115 A middle-aged patient complains of persistent nasal obstruction but no nasal discharge. This might be due to

A   diabetes mellitus
B   deviated nasal septum
C   enlarged adenoids
D   methylopa (Aldomet) therapy
E   prolonged use of a topical decongestant

116 Vestibular damage during treatment with streptomycin

A   is reversible
B   occurs more frequently in the elderly than in young adults
C   is particularly liable to occur in patients with liver disease
D   is associated with normal caloric tests of vestibular function
E   does not occur when the drug is administered orally

117 A patient presents with unilateral lower motor neurone facial paresis. The following statements are correct

A   If he has an ipsilateral acute exacerbation of chronic otitis media, an exploration of the middle ear cleft is urgently indicated
B   If the patient has acute otitis media, the facial paresis is likely to recover on antibiotic therapy alone
C   Hyperacusis is a recognized association
D   The cause of the paresis may be a localized cerebral cortical infarct
E   If the paresis is due to a herpes zoster infection of the geniculate ganglion, one would expect reduction or loss of taste sensation over the posterior third of the tongue

118 Carcinoma of the female breast

A   is less common than carcinoma of the uterine cervix
B   is unrelated to cystic hyperplasia of the breast
C   when intraductal in type may be associated with Paget's disease of the nipple
D   carries a worse prognosis when the axillary nodes show proliferation of plasma cells and histiocytes
E   is prone to metastasize to internal mammary lymph nodes

115

A	FALSE	I can't see why it should
B	TRUE	A well-recognized cause
C	FALSE	Not in this situation
D	TRUE	A well-recognized unwanted effect
E	TRUE	Remember this

116

A	FALSE	Irreversible
B	TRUE	Older patients are at much greater risk
C	FALSE	Liver disease is irrelevant — renal disease is certainly not
D	FALSE	Caloric tests are abnormal, indicating vestibular damage
E	TRUE	Very poor absorption

117

A	TRUE	Certainly. Otherwise there is likely to be permanent paresis
B	TRUE	This is correct
C	TRUE	Due to involvement of branch to stapedius
D	FALSE	I said a *lower* motor neurone paresis
E	FALSE	Glossopharyngeal nerve for posterior third of tongue. Loss of taste sensation over anterior two-thirds might be found if lesion involved facial nerve above the point at which chorda tympani leaves it

118

A	FALSE	It is more common
B	FALSE	The incidence of mammary carcinoma is greater in patients with cystic hyperplasia.
C	TRUE	A well recognized association
D	FALSE	Not so
E	TRUE	A common site of metastasis

119 The following conditions are associated in time with an increased risk of mucosal malignant change

A diverticular disease
B chronic duodenal ulcer
C familial polyposis coli

D villous papilloma
E Hirschsprung's disease

120 After major abdominal surgery (e.g. partial gastrectomy) the following metabolic changes would be expected to occur in the first four days postoperatively

A An increased utilization of glucose
B A reduction in the amount of sodium excreted in the urine
C A decrease in the circulating free fatty acid concentration

D An increased excretion of potassium in the urine
E An increase in oxygen consumption

121 Recognized complications of hiatal hernia include

A iron deficiency anaemia

B episodes of retrosternal pain

C fibrous stricture of the lower oesophagus
D persistent hiccups
E low serum vitamin B_{12} concentration

122 Hypokalaemia is a recognized complication of

A infestation with round worms
B a villous papilloma of the lower part of the large intestine
C phaeochromocytoma of the adrenal
D an α-cell tumour of the pancreas

E the chronic abuse of purgatives

119

A	FALSE	Does not occur
B	FALSE	Certainly does not occur
C	TRUE	May be multiple primaries. Screen close relatives of patients with polyposis coli
D	TRUE	Well recognized
E	FALSE	Not reported

120

A	FALSE	Glucose utilization is reduced
B	TRUE	Sodium retention occurs
C	FALSE	Circulating FFA levels rise — fat is the major energy substrate here
D	TRUE	A feature of the catabolic state that follows surgery
E	TRUE	This is known to occur

121

A	TRUE	And very easy (but remember that patients with hiatal hernias can also have asymptomatic caecal carcinomas)
B	TRUE	May mimic myocardial infarction — reflux oesophagitis; oesophageal spasm. There may be secondary ECG changes. Relieved by antacids and/or antispasmodics (including GTN)
C	TRUE	A recognized complication
D	FALSE	Not recognized
E	FALSE	No relationship

122

A	FALSE	Not to my knowledge
B	TRUE	A well-recognized cause of potassium depletion
C	FALSE	Not reported
D	TRUE	Zollinger–Ellison syndrome — due to the profuse diarrhoea that often occurs in these patients. Also seen, for the same reason, in 'vipomas' (tumours secreting vasoactive intestinal peptides)
E	TRUE	Must be remembered. Seen in anorexia nervosa

123 When a kidney is transplanted into a suitable recipient and functions well

A   hypertensive recipients may become normotensive
B   the recipient becomes more anaemic
C   if acute rejection occurs lymphocytes invade the graft
D   the thymus gland enlarges
E   the lymph nodes adjacent to the graft enlarge

124 A sixty-year-old lady is admitted to hospital with a six-week history of painless progressive jaundice. Her urine is dark and her stools clay coloured, and her gall bladder is palpable on abdominal examination. The serum bilirubin is 308 μmol/l (18 mg/100 ml)

A   A serum alkaline phosphatase concentration of 45 iu/l is consistent with this clinical picture
B   An oral cholecystogram is likely to give useful diagnostic information
C   It would be expected that her urinary excretion of urobilinogen would be increased
D   The absence of pain excludes a malignant lesion
E   The patient is likely to complain of considerable itching of the skin

125 Seminoma is a malignant neoplasm that

A   rarely metastasizes
B   carries a better prognosis after treatment than teratoma of the testis
C   may be associated with maldescent of the testis
D   responds to radiotherapy
E   characteristically presents with pain in the testis

123

A	TRUE	This can occur
B	FALSE	Likely to be the reverse
C	TRUE	A characteristic feature
D	FALSE	This does not occur
E	FALSE	Neither does this

124

A	FALSE	A normal alkaline phosphatase would certainly *not* be consistent with what is clearly obstructive jaundice
B	FALSE	Certainly not with a serum bilirubin as high as this
C	FALSE	No. Not with obstructive jaundice
D	FALSE	This is not so. Nor would the presence of pain. The picture described very strongly suggests malignant disease; probably carcinoma of head of pancreas
E	TRUE	Yes. This can be a most distressing feature. May be relieved by cholestyramine

125

A	FALSE	Metastasis is common — regional lymph nodes and also lungs etc.
B	TRUE	This is a fact
C	TRUE	Should be well known — incidence of malignancy in undescended (particularly intra-abdominal) testis is high
D	TRUE	The tumour is radiosensitive
E	FALSE	This is not a characteristic feature. A painless swelling is the usual presentation

126 In a patient with acute pancreatitis

A alcoholism is a recognized association

B serial estimations of the serum calcium concentration should be performed following admission

C acute renal failure is a recognized complication
D immediate laparotomy is indicated
E jaundice is a recognized feature

127 Infection of the genito-urinary tract by *M. tuberculosis*

A is a primary infection by the organism

B characteristically causes pain in the affected kidney

C is typically accompanied by pyuria with sterile urine on routine culture

D should not be treated until the organism is cultured

E causes frequency of micturition only when the bladder is directly involved

128 Recognized features of untreated carcinoma of the prostate include

A raised serum acid phosphatase activity
B rectal bleeding
C testicular atrophy
D fibrinolysins in the serum

E prostatic infection

126

A	TRUE	Well recognized (responsible in 8 to 75% of cases, depending on the population studied). Mechanism not fully understood
B	TRUE	Hypocalcaemia well known, may cause tetany. Due partly to fixation of calcium by fatty acids in areas of fat necrosis and partly to high circulating glucagon levels (experimentally, glucagon causes hypocalcaemia)
C	TRUE	Also well recognized
D	FALSE	Conservative treatment advised in acute phase
E	TRUE	Causes include obstruction of terminal common duct as it traverses oedematous pancreas, exacerbation of associated biliary tract disease and alcoholic liver disease

127

A	FALSE	A blood-borne infection, usually seeded at the time of the initial infection
B	FALSE	Symptoms are often lacking, even with advanced lesions. Backache is uncommon
C	TRUE	A typical feature. Although the pyuria is sometimes low grade, renal tuberculosis must always be excluded in the presence of sterile pyuria (also occurs in analgesic nephropathy)
D	FALSE	It takes about 6 weeks to culture the organism. Treatment may be given on the basis of clinical picture and finding of AFB on microscopy of early morning urine
E	FALSE	Symptoms of an irritable bladder are well recognized in renal tuberculosis

128

A	TRUE	Very easy
B	FALSE	Not recognized
C	FALSE	Not recognized
D	TRUE	Plasminogen activator, e.g. urokinase; streptokinase, may be released endogenously from activator – rich neoplastic tissue such as prostatic carcinoma, particularly if metastatic. Leads to a primary fibrinolytic disorder
E	FALSE	Not recognized

129 A fistula in the right iliac fossa is a recognized complication of

A   Crohn's disease
B   gastric ulcer
C   ulcerative colitis
D   tubo-ovarian infection
E   carcinoma of the caecum

130 In Crohn's disease

A   the risk of subsequent mucosal malignant change is greater than in ulcerative colitis
B   anal lesions are a recognized feature
C   the demonstration of vitamin B_{12} malabsorption indicates involvement of the jejunum
D   eye signs indistinguishable from those complicating ulcerative colitis may occur
E   controlled trials have shown that steroid therapy is beneficial

131 A forty-seven-year-old housewife presents with a three week history of pain in the right shoulder. There was no precipitating trauma and the pain is getting worse, occasionally waking her at night. The pain is felt over the point of the shoulder and spreads halfway down the outer side of the upper arm. She has found it progressively more difficult to reach above the head with the right arm. In this patient

A   if a 'painful arc' can be described it will be found during the course of flexion of the shoulder
B   pain felt on the outer aspect of the upper arm is due to a traction injury of the deltoid insertion
C   a diagnosis of 'frozen shoulder' is appropriate
D   if an X-ray of the shoulder reveals a deposit of calcified material in the region of the supraspinatus tendon, an attempt should be made to aspirate this
E   the demonstration of weakness of the supraspinatus muscle would suggest the possibility of a disorder affecting the subscapular nerve

129

A	TRUE
B	FALSE
C	FALSE
D	FALSE
E	TRUE

A very elementary level of knowledge

130

A   FALSE   Greater risk than in normal individuals but considerably less than in ulcerative colitis

B   TRUE   Anal, perianal and perirectal abscesses and fissure are often the presenting complaint

C   FALSE   Vitamin B_{12} absorbed in the ileum

D   TRUE   Iritis, irido-cyclitis etc. Less common than in ulcerative colitis but are non-specific

E   FALSE   This has not yet been shown

131

A   FALSE   The painful area is in abduction

B   FALSE   Traction injury of the deltoid insertion is not a recognized entity

C   FALSE   A 'frozen shoulder' is one with *no* gleno-brachial movements, active or passive

D   TRUE   Attempted aspiration is successful in 80% of patients and dramatically relieves symptoms

E   FALSE   Supraspinatus is supplied by the suprascapular nerve

132 Osteogenic sarcoma

A   is characterized histologically by the primary formation of osteoid
B   is a recognized complication of Paget's disease of bone (osteitis deformans)
C   is characteristically associated with hypercalcaemia
D   may metastasize to other bones
E   may be osteolytic

133 In a patient with prolapse of the lumbo-sacral (L5/S1) intervertebral disk and right-sided sciatica

A   absence of the right knee jerk would be expected
B   a complaint of urinary incontinence of rapid onset would be an absolute indication for urgent exploration of the spinal cord
C   the demonstration of diminished sensation to light touch and pinprick on the inner side of the right calf would be consistent with the diagnosis
D   scoliosis of the lumbar spine, demonstrated on physical examination, is structural in nature
E   the most effective initial treatment is the application of a plaster of Paris body cast so that the patient may remain as active as possible

134 Following an injury to the knee in a twenty-three-year-old man, flexion is free but there is inability to extend the knee through the last five degrees of movement. These findings would be consistent with

A   lateral dislocation of the patella
B   torn meniscus
C   osteochondral fracture of a femoral condyle
D   cyst of the lateral cartilage
E   a loose body in the knee joint

132

A	TRUE	This is so
B	TRUE	Well recognized. Most cases of osteogenic sarcoma occurring in older patients do so in pre-existing Paget's disease (incidence probably one per 4,000 Paget patients per year)
C	FALSE	Hypercalcaemia occurs only very rarely
D	TRUE	Well recognized
E	TRUE	Bone destruction or bone formation may predominate

133

A	FALSE	These signs indicate L4 root involvement which is impossible with lumbo-sacral disk prolapse
B	TRUE	The one indication for urgent exploration is loss of bladder sphincter control
C	FALSE	The dermatome described is appropriate to the L4 nerve root. See comment on **A**
D	FALSE	The scoliosis is postural, not structural
E	FALSE	The best initial treatment is bed rest with analgesics

134

A	FALSE	No
B	TRUE	A typical feature
C	TRUE	Also a typical feature
D	FALSE	No way
E	TRUE	Yes, often with other signs

135 A seventy-five-year-old patient with intertrochanteric fracture of the femur

A would be seen on clinical examination to lie with the affected leg internally rotated
B would best be treated by traction in a Thomas splint for at least eight weeks
C faces the possibility of non-union of the fracture because of damage to the blood supply to the femoral head
D has sustained an injury which is known to be one of the commonest causes of fat embolism
E carries an abnormally high risk of venous thrombo-embolism

136 A sixty-five-year-old woman has been found to have severe senile (post-menopausal) osteoporosis. In this patient

A appropriate histological examination of a bone biopsy from the iliac crest will show abnormally large amounts of unmineralized bone matrix
B the serum calcium will characteristically be normal
C there is an increased susceptibility to osteoarthrosis of the hip joints
D radiological examination of the dorso-lumbar spine will be unlikely to show any abnormality
E treatment with vitamin D by injection will lead to demonstrable improvement in the condition within six months

137 Suxamethonium (Scoline)

A is extremely irritant to the tissues in the event of extravenous injection
B is a competitive blocker of neuro-muscular transmission
C has a prolonged action in liver failure
D is known to cause muscle pain post-operatively
E may cause bradycardia when administered intermittently

135

A	FALSE	The leg is *always* externally rotated in this injury
B	FALSE	Treatment is aimed at mobilizing the patient as rapidly as possible. Operative fixation of the fracture is therefore indicated so that the patient can be out of bed within 2 days and walking within 2 weeks
C	FALSE	Non-union of intertrochanteric fracture is virtually unknown
D	FALSE	Fat embolism in association with isolated fractures of the upper femur is virtually unknown
E	TRUE	The incidence of venous thrombosis in elderly females with upper femoral fractures is over 40%

136

A	FALSE	Unmineralized matrix is a feature of osteomalacia but not osteoporosis
B	TRUE	The serum calcium is normal in osteoporosis
C	FALSE	There is no known correlation between osteoporosis and osteoarthrosis
D	FALSE	The spine is almost invariably affected — this may be the reason the diagnosis was made
E	FALSE	Vitamin D is not known to improve the clinical symptoms or the radiological or histological parameters in senile osteoporosis

137

A	FALSE	Non-irritant
B	FALSE	It is the non-depolarizing agents such as gallamine triethiodide that compete with acetyl choline for receptor sites on the motor end-plate. Depolarizing agents such as suxamethonium produce sustained depolarization of the motor end-plate rendering the tissues incapable of responding to transmitter
C	TRUE	This is so
D	TRUE	Well recognized. Can be quite severe
E	TRUE	May also cause transient hypertension

138 Post-operative jaundice may be causally related to

A surgery on the biliary tract
B pre-medication with Omnopon
C blood transfusion
D the repeated use of Halothane as an anaesthetic agent

E a long anaesthetic employing nitrous oxide

139 Carcinoma of the uterine cervix

A is characteristically squamous in type
B is preceded by a preinvasive stage which typically lasts for only a few months
C occurs more commonly in nulliparous than in multiparous patients
D may lead to ureteric obstruction

E characteristically metastasizes to the superficial inguinal lymph nodes

140 The following statements concerning the vagina are correct

A The upper part of the posterior wall alone is related directly to the peritoneal cavity
B Its wall contains mucus—secreting glands

C Its lateral fornix is closely related to the ureter

D the sphincter vaginae is a part of the levator ani muscle
E The glycogen content of the vaginal epithelium is directly related to the level of oestrogenic hormone

138

A	TRUE	Of course
B	FALSE	Of course not
C	TRUE	Elementary
D	TRUE	Typically Halothane jaundice appears after repeated, often short, exposures
E	FALSE	Never

139

A	TRUE	Obviously this is so
B	FALSE	The preinvasive stage is much longer than a few months
C	FALSE	More common in multiparous patients
D	TRUE	Correct. Remember the anatomical relations of the terminal portions of the ureters
E	FALSE	It certainly does not. Again, remember your anatomy

140

A	TRUE	Only the upper one-fourth of the posterior wall is so related
B	FALSE	Lined by mucous membrane, but no mucus—secreting glands therein
C	TRUE	As the terminal portions of the ureters approach the bladder they run close to the lateral fornices and they usually enter the bladder in front of the vagina
D	TRUE	This is so
E	TRUE	Correct

141 In pregnancy there is

A   increased gastric acidity

B   increased gastric motility
C   increased liability to peptic ulceration

D   slower emptying of the gall bladder

E   an increased tendency to gastro-oesophageal reflux

142 The climacteric is characteristically associated with

A   a reduced urinary excretion of follicle stimulating hormone
B   a reduced urinary oestrogen output
C   a decreased karyo-pyknotic index in the vaginal smear
D   an increase in the number of basal cells in a scrape smear taken from the cervix
E   a reduction in the serum cholesterol concentration

143 Certain changes occur in the constituents of the peripheral blood in pregnancy which affect the interpretation of laboratory reports. During a normal pregnancy

A   the serum cholesterol concentration rises
B   the haemoglobin concentration falls
C   the serum protein bound iodine concentration falls
D   the blood urea concentration rises
E   the erythrocyte sedimentation rate is accelerated

141

A	FALSE	Acid secretion, fasting or after histamine, is considerably reduced during most of pregnancy
B	FALSE	Gastric tone and motility are decreased in pregnancy
C	FALSE	Well known. Peptic ulceration rare and established ulcers tend to heal. Not due solely to reduced acid secretion — increased mucous secretion (protective) under influence of oestrogens
D	TRUE	The gallbladder shares the general smooth muscle atony of the gut
E	TRUE	Persistent regurgitation of gastric acid — may be associated with particularly slow gastric emptying

142

A	FALSE	Increased (feedback)
B	TRUE	Ovarian failure
C	TRUE	Secondary to oestrogen deficiency
D	TRUE	See comment on C
E	FALSE	The reverse, if anything

143

A	TRUE	This is correct
B	TRUE	This occurs, due to haemodilution, and is physiological
C	FALSE	PBI rises, due to increased levels of thyroxine-binding globulin (also with oral contraceptives containing oestrogen)
D	FALSE	The blood urea falls
E	TRUE	The ESR rises at an early stage and must be interpreted with caution during pregnancy

144 Polyhydramnios is a recognized association of

A   anencephalus in the fetus

B   maternal cardiac disease

C   maternal diabetes mellitus

D   Potter's syndrome (renal agenesis) in the fetus

E   uniovular twin pregnancy

145 The following statements regarding tuberculosis of the female genital tract are correct

A   The majority of cases are diagnosed in patients complaining of childlessness
B   Secondary amenorrhoea is a characteristic presenting symptom
C   In most cases involvement of the genital tract occurs at or close to puberty
D   The most reliable method of diagnosing genital tuberculosis is by guinea-pig inoculation of endometrium taken in the second half of the menstrual cycle
E   Fertility will be restored to normal after adequate anti-tuberculous therapy

146 The following changes during the menstrual cycle suggest that ovulation has taken place

A   mid-cycle pain in the iliac fossa region
B   fern pattern in dried cervical mucus
C   a rise in basal body temperature

D   an increase in the clear mucus secretion by the cervix
E   the presence of red cells in the cervical mucus

144

A	TRUE	Anencephaly prevents the fetus from swallowing the liquor
B	FALSE	Even severe maternal cardiac disease with generalized oedema does not increase the volume of liquor
C	TRUE	Not closely correlated with the degree of diabetic control achieved
D	FALSE	Renal agenesis prevents the fetus from circulating liquor through the urine
E	TRUE	Binovular twin pregnancy is not associated with polyhydramnios whereas uniovular twin pregnancy is

145

A	TRUE	Genital tuberculosis is usually asymptomatic
B	FALSE	The menstrual cycle is usually normal although they may develop menorrhagia
C	TRUE	Primary infection usually occurs in late childhood
D	TRUE	All other methods of diagnosis have a high failure rate
E	FALSE	Less than one-quarter of patients will be able to conceive following genital tract tuberculosis

146

A	TRUE	Mid-cycle pain is commonly associated with ovulation
B	FALSE	Ferning occurs before ovulation and not afterwards
C	TRUE	A rise in basal body temperature occurs because of the increased progesterone concentration
D	TRUE	The mucus becomes more profuse at the time of ovulation
E	TRUE	Red cells appear in the cervical mucus at the time of ovulation

147 The composition of amniotic fluid alters as normal pregnancy advances in the following ways

A   the pH rises
B   The glucose concentration falls
C   the sodium concentration rises
D   the oestriol concentration rises

E   the oestradiol concentration rises

148 The human fetus can be adversely affected by the following maternal situations

A   rubella infection in early pregnancy

B   heparin administered intravenously during the antenatal period
C   cigarette smoking
D   heroin addiction
E   streptomycin administered during pregnancy

149 During a normal menstrual cycle

A   proliferative changes in the endometrium follow ovulation

B   the plasma progesterone concentration rises following ovulation
C   the average menstrual blood loss is 400 ml per cycle
D   ovulation is dependent upon an intact hypothalamic pituitary portal circulation
E   the menstrual loss is normally fluid because of the presence of fibrinolysins in the endometrium

147

A	FALSE	There tends to be a slight fall in pH
B	TRUE	There is a progressive fall in concentration
C	FALSE	It falls progressively
D	TRUE	Rises progressively. Depressed if infant is *severely* affected by rhesus haemolytic disease
E	FALSE	Oestriol is the only oestrogen present in the amniotic fluid in any substantial amount

148

A	TRUE	Frequency of fetal malformation 10–15%. Organs involved include eye, ear, brain and heart
B	FALSE	Heparin is safe
C	TRUE	Small babies
D	TRUE	Very bad
E	TRUE	Can cause deafness and vestibular dysfunction in the child

149

A	FALSE	Proliferative (follicular) phase is pre-ovulatory. Post-ovulatory phase is secretory (luteal) (progestational) phase
B	TRUE	Secreted by corpus luteum
C	FALSE	Average blood loss normally about 120 ml
D	TRUE	Of course. Secretion of gonadotrophins from pituitary under influence of hypothalamic releasing hormones
E	TRUE	This is a fact

150 A patient presents with vaginal blood loss and abdominal pain at the tenth week of pregnancy

A   She is having an antepartum haemorrhage

B   Digital vaginal examination should be performed

C   If the immunological pregnancy test is positive to a dilution of 1 in 20 then a diagnosis of hydatidiform mole can be made

D   A previous history of three spontaneous abortions between the eighth and twelfth week of pregnancy would suggest a diagnosis of cervical incompetence

E   If this pregnancy continues to term there are no increased risks to this fetus compared with a pregnancy not associated with early bleeding

150

A FALSE She is threatening to abort. Antepartum haemorrhage is bleeding after the 28th week of pregnancy
B TRUE Vaginal examination must be performed to diagnose whether this is a threatened or an inevitable abortion
C FALSE Hydatidiform mole can only be suspected when the pregnancy test is positive to a dilution much higher than 1 in 20
D FALSE A previous history of abortion between the 12th and 20th week of pregnancy would be required to suggest a diagnosis of cervical incompetence
E FALSE There is increased mortality for the fetus when the pregnancy has been associated with early bleeding

Index to Questions

(The numbers given are those of the questions and are not page numbers).

Acholuric jaundice, *see* spherocytosis, hereditary
Acromegaly, 82
Adenoidectomy, indications for, 113
Alcoholism, 50
Alkaline phosphatase activity, serum — elevation of, 87
Alopecia, *see* diffuse hair loss
Altitude, effects of, 13, 15
Amniotic fluid, 147
    polyhydramnios, 144
Amyloidosis, secondary, 90
Ankylosing spondylitis, 92
Anorexia nervosa, features of, 79
Appendix, the —
    anatomy of, 30
Arterial blood —
    carbon dioxide tension, factors determining in normal subjects, 17
    oxygen content, 14
    partial pressure of carbon dioxide, 15
Arthritis, 95
Arthropathy, associated skin diseases, 3
Atrial fibrillation and mitral stenosis, 57

Baby, newborn —
    normal, 36
    respiratory distress syndrome in, 35
'Bends', the, 13
Biguanide drugs, 23
Blisters, 6
Breast, carcinoma of, 118
Bronchial carcinoma, 62
Bronchitis —
    acute viral, 60
    chronic, respiratory failure in, 63

Carbon dioxide —
    partial pressure in arterial blood, 15
    tension in arterial blood, factors determining in normal subjects, 17

Carcinoma —
    cutaneous manifestations of, 7
    of breast, 118
    of bronchus, as occupational hazard, 62
    of gastrointestinal tract, 119
    of large intestine, 32
    of prostate, 128
    of uterine cervix, 139
    of vocal cord, 114
Carpal tunnel compression syndrome, 101
Cell regeneration, 29
Cerebrospinal fluid, 97
Cervical sympathetic, paralysis of, 96
Cholestatic jaundice, drug induced, 21
Climacteric, 142
Clubbing of fingers, causes, 59
'Compensation' neurosis, 47
Constipation, as a presenting feature, 73
Contraceptives, oral —
    unwanted effects, 81
Coronary thrombosis, aftercare, 56
Craniopharyngioma, 41
Creatine phosphokinase, *see* creatine phosphotransferase
Creatine phosphotransferase, 91
Crohn's disease, features, 130
Cushing's syndrome, features, 84
Cystic fibrosis, 37

Delusions, 46
Dementia, 49
Depression —
    endogenous, 48
    late onset depressive psychosis, 51
Diabetes mellitus —
    increased insulin resistance in, 80
    ocular changes in, 108
    therapy, 23
Digoxin therapy, contraindications to, 54
Diplopia, 105
Drowning, 13
Drugs, unwanted effects of —
    oral contraceptives, 81

Drugs, unwanted effects of — (contd.)
    propranolol, 22
    streptomycin, 116
    suxamethonium, 137
    various, 19, 20, 21

Earache, intermittent, 111
Emphysema and chronic bronchitis, respiratory failure in, 63
Encephalopathy, portal-systemic — precipitating factors, 71
Enuresis, nocturnal, 42
Enzyme activity in serum —
    alkaline phosphatase, 87
    creatine phosphotransferase, 91
Erythema nodosum, 1

Facial paresis, lower motor neurone, 117
Femur, intertrochanteric fracture of, 135
Fetus, adverse effects on, 148
Fibrosing alveolitis, features of, 61
Fistula in right iliac fossa, causes, 129
Fungal infection, cutaneous — predisposing factors, 2

Gastric emptying, factors influencing, 72
Gastrointestinal tract —
    carcinoma of, 32, 119
    changes in pregnancy, 141
    drug-induced ulceration of, 20
Glandular fever, 70
Glaucoma, acute (narrow angle), 106

Haematuria —
    in childhood, 33
    microscopic, 76
Hair loss, diffuse, 5
Heberden's nodes, 93
Hiatal hernia, complications and features, 121
Hodgkin's disease, 31
Hyperglycaemia, see diabetes mellitus
Hyperthyroidism —
    eye disease in, 109
    therapy, 85
Hypoglycaemia, 83
Hypokalaemia, 24, 122
Hyponatraemia, 16
Hypothyroidism, pathological changes in, 27

Infectious mononucleosis, see glandular fever
Intervertebral disk prolapse, 133
Irritable bowel syndrome, 74

Jaundice —
    cholestatic (drug induced), 21
    obstructive, 124
    post-operative, 138

Kidney transplantation, 123
Knee, injuries to, 134

Large intestine, carcinoma of, 32
Leucocytosis, polymorphonuclear, 66
Leukoplakia, oral, 8
Liver disease, advanced —
    portal-systemic encephalopathy in, 71
Lumbar puncture, see cerebrospinal fluid

Manic states, therapy, 52
Measles, 43
Menarché, the, 44
Menstrual cycle, normal, 149
Mitral stenosis and atrial fibrillation, 57
Motor neurone disease, 99
Mucoviscidosis, see cystic fibrosis
Myocardial infarction, see coronary thrombosis
Myocardium, normal ventricular, 58

Nasal obstruction, causes, 115
Neck stiffness, 98
Nephrotic syndrome, 75

Obesity, features of, 88
Occupational hazards —
    bronchial carcinoma, 62
Osteogenic sarcoma, 132
Osteoporosis, senile, 136
Otosclerosis, 112
Ovulation, changes associated with, 146
Oxygen, content of arterial blood, 14

'Painful shoulder' syndrome, 131
Pancreatitis, acute, 126
Pancytopenia, 65
Parkinson's disease, 102
Pathogens, faecal spread of, 9
Pericarditis, 55
Pernicious anaemia (Addisonian), 28, 69
Petit mal, features of, 103
Pleural effusion, blood-stained, 64
Pneumonitis, acute viral, 60
Poliomyelitis, vaccines against, 10
Polycystic renal disease, 77
Polycythraemia rubra vera, 67
Polyhydramnios, 144
Potassium depletion (see also hypokalaemia), drug induced, 24
Pregnancy —
    adverse effects on fetus, 148
    changes in amniotic fluid composition during, 147
    changes in peripheral blood during, 143
    effects on gastrointestinal tract, 141
    polyhydramnios, 144
    urinary infection in, 78
    vaginal blood loss in, 150

Propranolol, unwanted effects, 22
Prostate, carcinoma of, 128
Protein-bound iodine, factors affecting, 89
Pruritus, 4
Pulse, collapsing, 53

Renal failure —
   acidaemia in, 15
   drug therapy in, 25
   due to polycystic renal disease, 77
Respiratory distress syndrome of the newborn, 35
Respiratory failure, due to chronic bronchitis and emphysema, 63
Reticulosis —
   cutaneous manifestations of, 7
   Hodgkin's disease, 31
Rickets, nutritional —
   features, 38

Salicylate poisoning, 26
Schizophrenia, 45
Sciatica, 133
Scoline, *see* suxamethonium
Scurvy, 86
Seminoma of testis, 125
Sjögren's syndrome, 94
Spherocytosis, hereditary, (acholuric jaundice), 68
Squint, in childhood, 104
Streptococci, haemolytic, 140

Streptomycin, causing vestibular damage, 116
Stridor, 34
Sulphonamides, causing renal failure, 19
Sulphonylurea drugs, 23
Surgery, metabolic response to, 120
Suxamethonium, 137

Tetanus, 39
Thyroid eye disease, 109
Thyrotoxicosis, *see* hyperthyroidism
Tuberculin, 11
Tuberculosis —
   genitourinary, 127
   of female genital tract, 145
Typhoid fever, 12

Ulceration, gastrointestinal —
   drug-induced, 20
   in pregnancy, 141
Ulnar nerve, complete interruption of, 18
Urinary infection, in pregnancy, 78
Uterine cervix, carcinoma of, 139
Uveitis, anterior, 107

Vagina, anatomy of, 140
Vaginal bleeding during pregnancy, 150
Vestibular damage due to streptomycin, 116
Visual fields, abnormalities of, 100
Visual loss, sudden onset of, 110
Vocal cord, carcinoma of, 114

General Index

Amended scores, 32, 34—6
   printout, 51—3

Calculation of scores, 24, 26, 33
Computer (*see also* Newcastle computer marking program) —
   English Electric KDF9, 24
   IBM 360/67, 26
   IBM 370/168, 27
   marking of MCQ, 23, 31—7
Correlation coefficients, viii, 26, 34—6, 41
   evaluation of questions, 40—1
   item analysis, 42—3
   point biserial, 42, 47, 51
   printout, 49—51
   product moment, 42
   revision of questions, 45—8

Document — reading machines (*see also* response sheets) —
   English Electric Lector, 24, 27, 29, 31, 33
   Opscan 17, 27, 28, 29, 31, 33
'Don't know' option, 4, 5, 24, 26, 27

English Electric Lector, 24, 27, 29, 31, 33
Erasive patient management problems, 2
Evaluation of MCQ, *see* multiple choice questions, evaluation

Feedback to examiners, 46

Grouped true/false questions, *see* multiple true/false questions

Hand-marked answer sheets, 23
Hand-marking of MCQ —
   multiple true/false, 30
   one-from-five, 37, 38
'Hidden bonus', 24

Indices of discrimination, viii, 26, 34—6, 40, 41
   evaluation of questions, 40—41
   item analysis, 42—3
   printout, 49—51
   revision of questions, 45—8
Instructions to candidates, 54—5

Items, viii, 4, 5, 7
   analysis, 42—3
   response statistics, 49—51
   revision of, 45—8
   wording, 15—21

Machine — marking of MCQ —
   multiple true/false, 31—7
   one-from-five, 38
Marker questions, 38, 44—5
Marking of MCQ, *see* multiple choice questions, marking
Marking program, *see* Newcastle computer marking program
Missing-link questions, 2
Modified essay questions, 2
Multiple choice questions, evaluation, 40—3
   discrimination when hand marked, 43
   item analysis, 42—3
   of individual questions, 41
   phi index, 42—3
Multiple choice questions, marking, 26—7, 30—9
   amended scores, 32, 34—6, 51—3
   calculation of scores, 24, 26, 33
   hand-marking of multiple true/false, 30
   machine marking of multiple true/false, 31—7
   of one-from-five questions, 37—8
   pass mark, setting, 38—9
   raw scores, 32, 33—6, 51—3
   short-scale mark conversion, 35, 37
   weighting of questions, 33—4
Multiple choice questions, revision, 44—8
   marker questions, 38, 44—5
   feedback to examiners, 46
Multiple choice questions, setting, 13—22
   double-barrelled items, 20
   mutually exclusive items, 19—20
   negatives, 20
   precision, 18—19
   setting a paper, 21—2
   special considerations for one-from-five, 21
   topics and content, 14—15
   wording, 15—18

Multiple choice questions, types, 1–12
   clinical problem-solving, 5, 6, 8, 9, 11, 12
   complex variants, 7, 11–12
   multiple true/false, 4–5, 7, 12
   one-from-five, 3–4, 5, 7
   yes/no alternative, 3
Multiple completion type of question, 7
Multiple true/false type of question, 4–5, 7, 12
   candidate responses, 23–9
   evaluation, 40–43
   marking, 30–37
   revision, 44–8
   setting, 14–22
Mutually exclusive items, 19–20

Newcastle computer marking program, vi, vii, 23, 29
   indices of discrimination, 26, 34–6, 40–43
   marking of multiple true/false questions, 31–8
   printout, 49–53
   question response statistics, 49–51
   ranked and unranked candidate lists, 51–3
   response sheets, 23–9

Objective examinations, 2
One-from-five type of question, 3–4, 5, 7
   candidate responses, 29
   evaluation, 43
   marking, 37–8
   setting, 21
Opscan 17, 27–9, 31, 33
Opscan sheets, 27–9, 31, 42, 51

Pass mark, setting, 38–9
Phi index (correlation), 42–3
Point biserial correlation coefficient, 42, 47, 51
Printout, 49–53
Product moment correlation coefficient, 42
Program, marking, *see* Newcastle computer marking program

Raw score, 32, 33–6, 51–3
Relationship analysis type of question, 7
Response sheets, 23–9
   hand-marked answer sheets, 23
   instructions to candidates, 54–5
   Lector sheets, 24–7, 29, 31, 42
   Opscan sheets, 27–9, 31, 42, 51
Responses (*see also* response sheets), viii, 23, 24, 26–7
Revision of MCQ, *see* Multiple choice questions, revision

Scoring of MCQ, *see* Multiple choice questions, marking
Setting of MCQ, *see* multiple choice questions, setting
Short scale mark conversion, 35, 37, 51
Standard score, 32–3, 51, 52
Stem, viii, 3, 4, 5, 7
   revision of stem, 45–8
   wording of stem, 15–21

Types of MCQ, *see* multiple choice questions, types

University of Newcastle upon Tyne, *see* Newcastle computer marking program

Weighting of questions, 33–4